It is recommended that only the Arasatma Breath sound elixirs be used when practicing the breath techniques. The elixirs were specifically received with this body of information and are included with the purchase of this book. They work in conjunction with the breaths, using the alchemical potencies of frequency incorporated within them. For an explanation of how sound elixirs function, see www. soundhealing.com.

- http://qr.spiritualjourneys.com/SevenBreathsofEternalLife.mp3

 Almine has created paintings that are supplementary to the information in Level II of the Arasatma Breaths. They can be used as a focus of meditation prior to doing the Breath techniques. The colors of the paintings embody the principles of each breath and match the colors that are visualized with the Breaths. To purchase the paintings visit:

- http://alminewisdom.com/collections/mystical-healing-art

The Sacred Breaths of Arasatma

Alchemical Breathing
Techniques of the Ancients

Almine

Mastering the Breaths of Eternal Life

Published by Spiritual Journeys LLC

First Edition July 2013

Copyright 2013

MAB 998 Megatrust
By Almine
Spiritual Journeys LLC
P.O. Box 300 Newport, Oregon 97365

US toll-free phone: 1-877-552-5646

www.spiritualjourneys.com

Cover Illustration - Charles Frizzell

Manufactured in the United States of America

ISBN 978-1-936926-64-0 Softcover

ISBN 978-1-936926-65-7 Adobe Reader

Table of Contents

Book II

Nevi-Satma – The Twelve Breaths of Proxy

Enhancing the Nutritional Frequency of Food

Book III

Ma-atma Suhat – The Breaths of Evolved Awareness

Appendices

Liability Disclaimer

Spiritual Journeys, LLC and/or Almine expressly disclaim any liability, loss, damage or injury in connection with the use of the Sacred Breaths of Arasatma. Almine is not a medical practitioner, nor does she practice medicine. Use of the breathing techniques is not intended to constitute medical advice or treatment. All persons with a medical condition (including pregnancy) are advised to consult with a physician or other qualified health provider prior to using the information in this book.

Directions are provided for the use of the Sacred Breaths of Arasatma per each level. Follow the directions as given, although specific postures may be modified for your own comfort and safety. For example, the use of pillows or positioning devices may be used to maintain proper body alignment or ease when performing the breaths.

Detoxification symptoms may be experienced following the breathing exercises. Drink plenty of water and rest as needed. Follow the guidelines and pre-requisites for each level.

Interdimensional Photo of Almine Writing

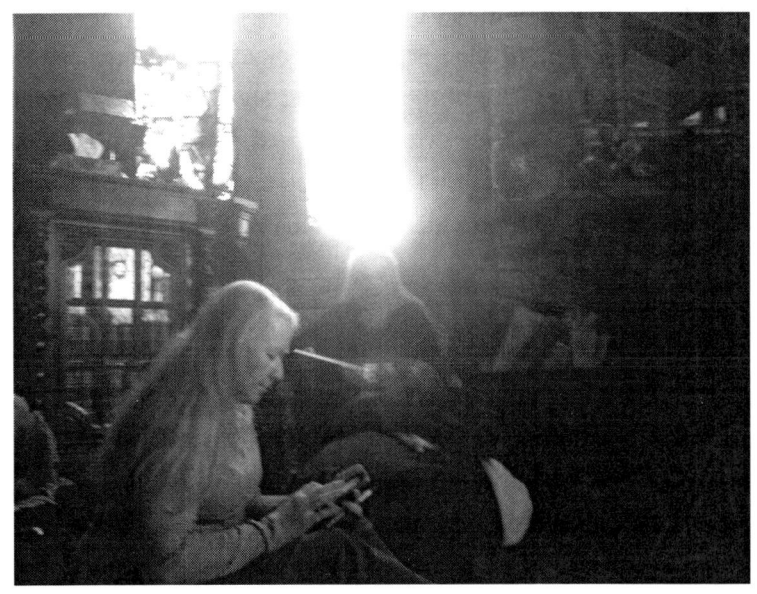

Photo taken by Donna, Canada

A ball of light appears around the Seer's writing. All books
are written by hand.

Photo of the Seer Almine

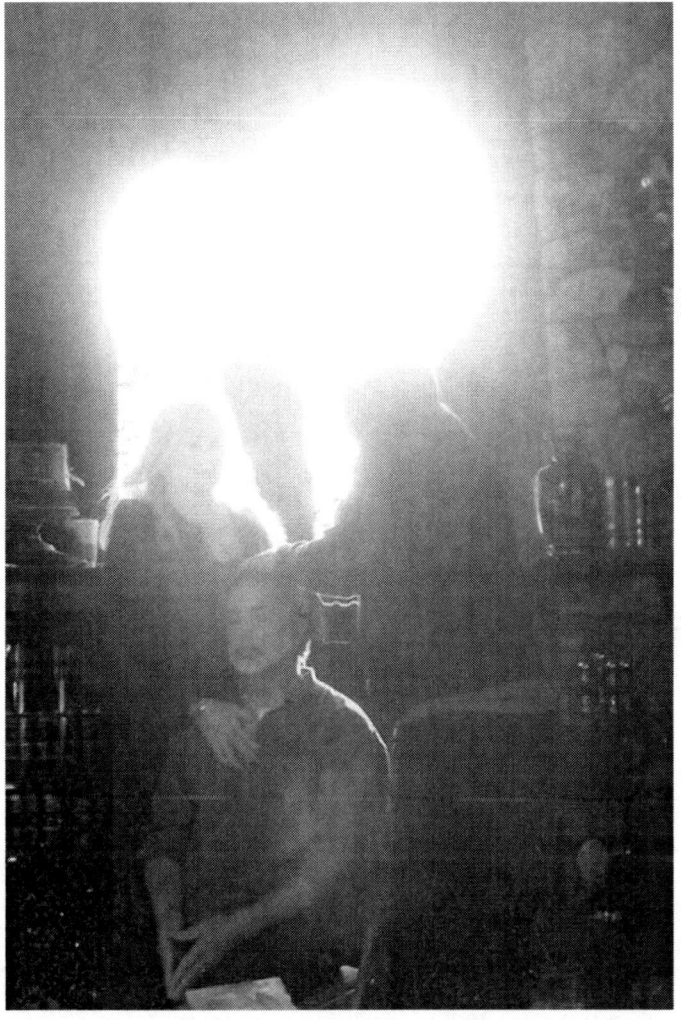

The Seer blesses a student in her class.

BOOK ONE

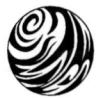

The Arasatma Breaths

The Seven Sacred Breaths of Eternal Life

Introduction to the Arasatma Breaths

When Ponce de Leon searched for the Fountain of Youth (also known as the Fountain of Life) among the native tribes of Florida, he did not realize that he was looking for the secret knowledge of breathing techniques. The tribe, known as the Montauk Indians, were the custodians of this sacred body of information. They dwelled on Montauk Island, New York, built pyramids and had leaders that were known as Paro (Pharaoh), which meant 'wisdom keeper'. As late as 1910, their pyramids could still be seen protruding from the sandy beaches.

The 7th breath of Arastama, moves like a fountain out of the top of the head and around the body, creating a dynamic balance between the three vehicles of experience: body, soul and spirit. This creates a closed system, a self-generating dynamo that can sustain youth and maintain health.

The two main causes of the energy leakages that cause aging, death and loss of conscious awareness are:

- The adversarial relationships between body, soul and spirit that creates mutual pillaging of resources.
- The shallow existence of physicality that uses only half the pranic tube as the channel for the flow of resources. The portion of pranic flow that is available is often blocked by unresolved issues that cause blockages of debris in the chakras (referred to in the New Testament, the Book of Revelation, as the seven seals).

The pranic tube, when used in its full capacity, should extend from the 10th chakra above the head, down through the crown and perineum, all the way into the ground (a hand length into the ground). Many enlightened races have cultivated a tail to ensure that the full capacity of the pranic tube is used.

The perineum is referred to as the gate of life and death. The pranic tube portion that is above this point is the portion used in living, the portion below it is the part used after death (in the soul world). When the gate is opened and the full pranic tube is used, life and death are combined and lived simultaneously. This opens up immortality, inter-dimensional capacities and reduces the need to eat and sleep.

From the Hidden Libraries of the Two Whales

Shabach harsta avunesvi klevi vasta pre-unet misavach heresvi minavich subahet aves-vastra misunet.

Long ago there walked a race of wise ones upon the Earth and among them were those with tails, known for their sacred power.

The Chakras of the Body

For descriptions of the Lahun chakra's specific function, see *The Ring of Truth.*

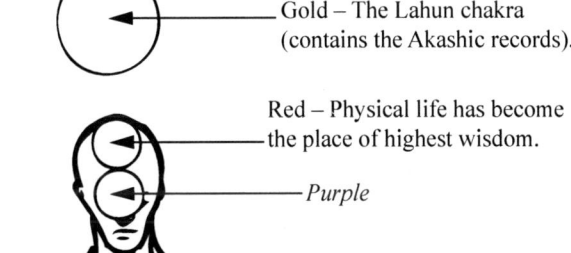

Gold – The Lahun chakra (contains the Akashic records).

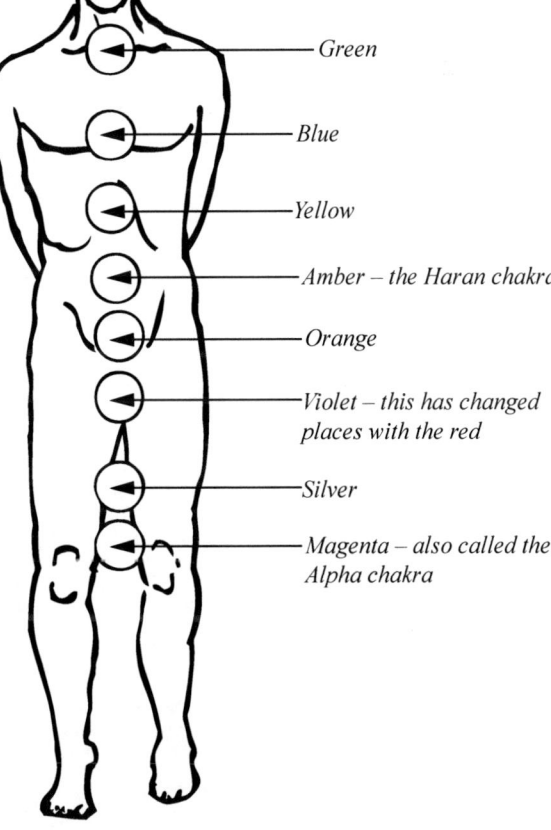

Red – Physical life has become the place of highest wisdom.

Purple

Green

Blue

Yellow

Amber – the Haran chakra

Orange

Violet – this has changed places with the red

Silver

Magenta – also called the Alpha chakra

The little known silver chakra contains a living library of Earth history. Anciently called the Braamish chakra, the word Braamin comes from there.

Transfigurations in the body have also led to the same large changes taking place in the chakra system.

The Fountain of Life

*There have been prophecies given that in
'The Time of Gathering', the Seven Breaths
of Eternal Life shall again be known among
men. Then shall the magic of life be restored.*

The Arasatma Breaths Level I

Opening the Channels of Prana

Guidelines for Level I

The first 4 breaths are done in a seated position with the spine straight and legs crossed. The remaining 3 breaths are done while lying down.

As you do the exercises, play the musical elixir that has been specifically created to accompany the Arasatma Breaths.

Some of the breaths include eye movements; these may be done with either your eyes closed or open, as preferred. Hands are held in a relaxed position for Level I.

For each of the exercises, the breaths should be repeated 12 times (the in- and out-breath count as one breath), except for Breath 6 which consists of 2 breaths for each cycle, making a total of 24 breaths.

When breathing for these exercises, draw the breath in (inhale) through the nose and blow the breath out (exhale) through the mouth.

For breaths 1 – 6, the breath circles within the body. Breath 7 circles outside the body.

You may wish to place the sigils that accompany these breaths in front of you to look at during the exercises.

These techniques facilitate the release of bodily toxins, so it is advisable that you increase your intake of water. You may also experience some heat and the release of emotions, as well as the appearance of images from your past either during the breaths or after them.

1. Atma seba uhut
The Breath of the Lion's Gate

I am an ever-new spontaneous expression of Infinite Existence.

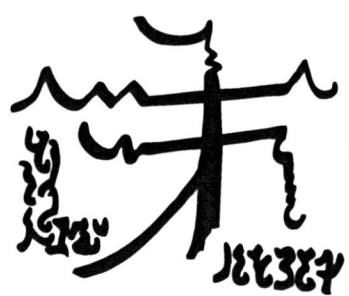

Breath:

- Sit with your spine straight and your legs crossed.
- The in-breath will cycle from the atlas joint (the place where the skull and the neck meet at the back of the neck), up the back of the skull, out of the crown (at the top of the head) and into the Lahun, or 10th chakra.
- The out-breath will cycle down from the Lahun, in through the crown chakra, and down the front of the skull and back to the atlas joint.
- Both the in- and out-breaths cycle inside the skull. Count to 5 on the in-breath and also on the out-breath.
- The breath flows like a stream, not as a line.

Eye movements:

• As you breathe in and out, your eyes will move to match the in- and out-breaths. Start with your eyes looking down towards the ground and as you breathe in, slowly raise your eyes upwards towards the sky. As you breathe out, slowly lower your eyes down again. The eyes may be open or closed, whichever is most comfortable. Repeat with each breath.

• Repeat this breathing pattern and eye movements for 12 cycles of in- and out-breaths.

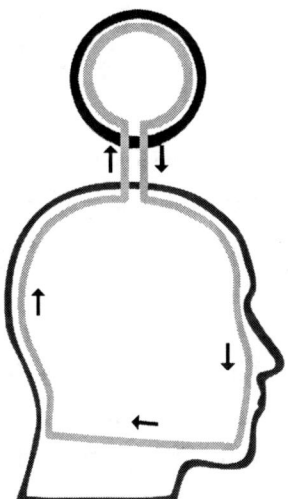

2. *Atma avi uhet nanastu*
The Breath of the Winged Ones

I am in surrendered stillness during automatic, proactive expression.

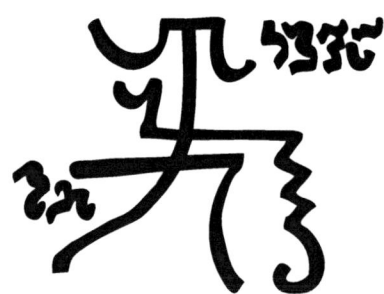

Breath:
- For this breath, only move the rib cage. Hold the rest of the torso (shoulders and abdomen) as still as possible.
- Breathe in deeply as you move the rib cage to the left. As you slowly breathe out, move the rib cage all the way to the right.
- When you have moved the rib cage all the way to the right, pause and breath in deeply, filling your lungs with air. Then move the rib cage to the left as you slowly breath out.
- When you have moved the rib cage to the left, pause and inhale deeply into the lungs and then slowly breath out again as you move the rib cage to the right.

Eye movements:
- For this breath the eyes look forward at all times.

- Repeat this for 12 cycles of in- and out-breaths.

Note: In Level I, Breath 2 flows the way a normal, deep breath would. It is however, synchronized with the movements of the rib cage. You breathe in when the rib cage is thrust all the way to the right or left, and breathe out as it moves across from side to side. There is no rotation of the breath or the rib cage, just the side to side movement.

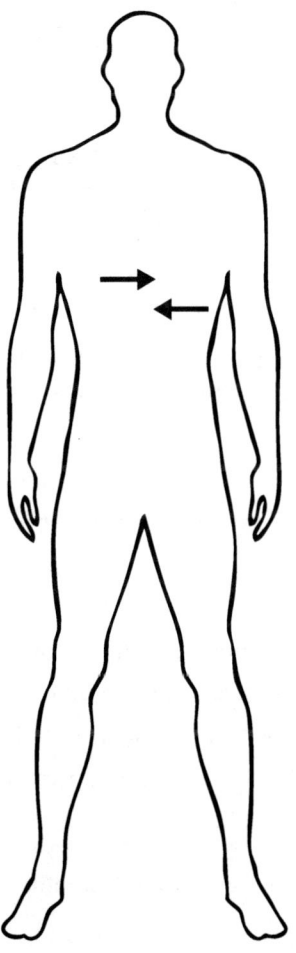

Breathe deeply into the lungs. The breath does not rotate. Only the rib cage moves from left to right and back again. It is important to isolate this movement as much as possible.

3. *Krihet atma unanes tuvi*
The Breath of Heaven and Earth

I embrace the changing expression of the fluid structure of my environment.

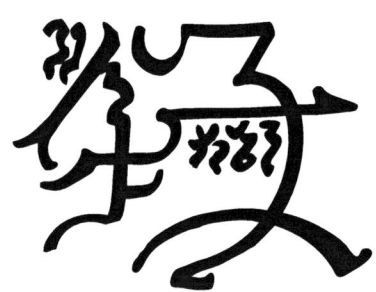

Breath:
- Starting at the midpoint directly above the pubic bone, breathe in deeply, moving the breath in a circular pattern up the right side of the body to the top of the abdomen (where the diaphragm is located).
- The breath is slowly blown out as it circles down the left side of the abdomen, back to the the midpoint above the pubic bone.

Eye movements:
- The eye movements match the rotation of the breath. Start by looking down as you breathe in and then rotate you eyes to the right and upward as you finish the in-breath. As you breathe out, rotate your eyes to the left and then downward as you complete the out-breath.

- Repeat for 12 cycles of in- and out-breaths.

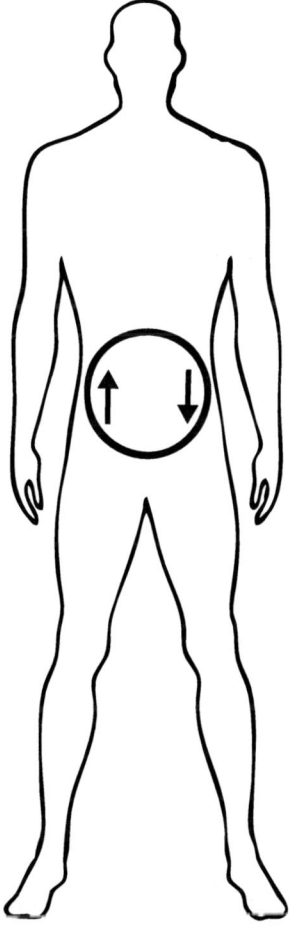

The Pranic Tube

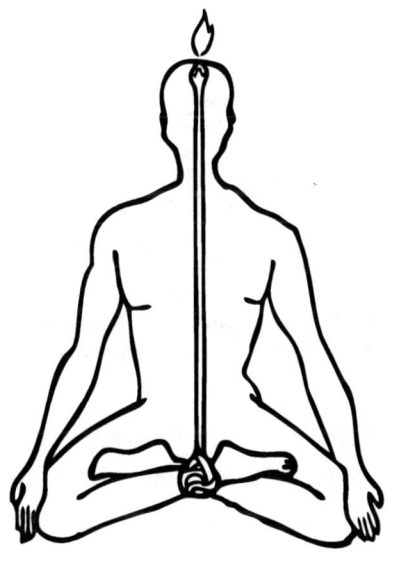

4. *Atma utu kranavesvi uhut*
The Breath of the Little Horn

I create my reality through the resonating emphases
of my heart.

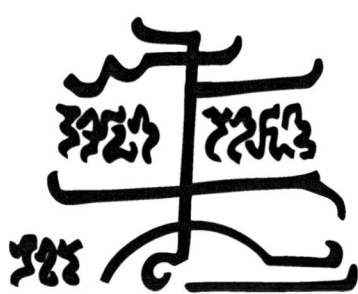

Breath:

- The pranic tube extends from the crown (at the top of the head) to the perineum (at the base of the spine). The diameter is the same as the circle created when your middle finger touches your thumb, tip to tip.
- Sages throughout the ages have known it to coil at the base of the spine like a serpent. The self-actualization (that which brings it into expression) of inner divinity requires that the coiled part of the pranic tube be straightened to yield its full use as the grounding rod of man. When straightened, it extends a hand length into the ground when you are standing.
- On the in-breath, draw in as much air as possible, breathing from the top of the crown to the navel. As this in-breath is drawn down the contracted panic tube, it becomes a power breath.
- Forcefully expel the breath down from the navel and out the base of the spine, blowing out all the blockages and debris of the past and straightening the pranic tube. With each breath, the pranic tube will become straighter until by breath 12, it will be extended fully into the ground.

Eye movements:

- For this posture the eyes remain looking forward.

- Repeat for 12 cycles of in- and out-breaths.

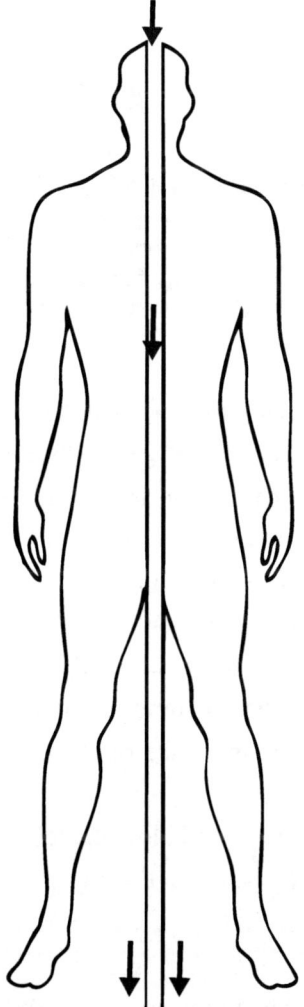

5. *Selva nechtasu atma karanu*
The Breath of the Fire Walk

I approach the newborn moment with the full awareness of adventurous discovery.

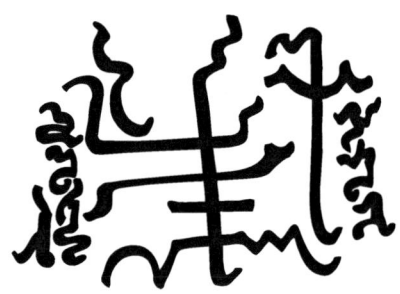

Breath:

- Lie down on your back with your hands in a relaxed position and your legs straight. There are no gaps between the in-breath and the out-breath and between the out-breath and the in-breath.
- Slowly and deeply, breathe in from a point one hand length below the left foot and draw the breath up the left leg, through the left hip and into the lower abdomen.
- In the middle of the abdomen, smoothly transition to a slow, deep out-breath and move the breath to the right hip and down the right leg, exiting out the bottom of the right foot and into the point, one hand length below it.
- Arc across to the same point below the left foot, moving the breath smoothly, with no gap between the out- and in-breath.

Eye movements:

- There are no specific eye movements for this breath.

- Repeat the exercise for 12 cycles of in- and out-breaths.

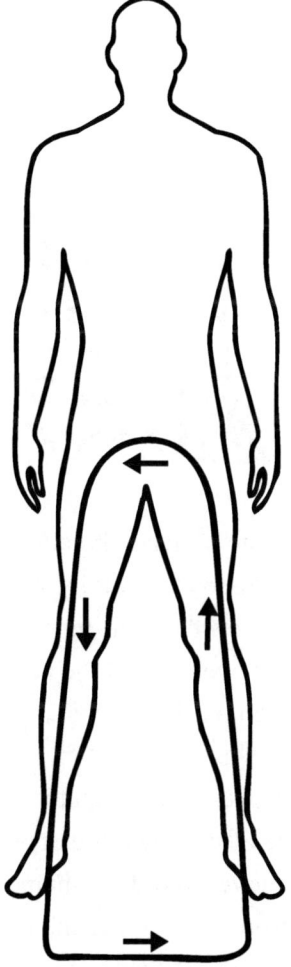

6. *Atma usu amara-uhet*
The Breath of the Divine Marriage

True peace is my constant companion through embracing unknowable change.

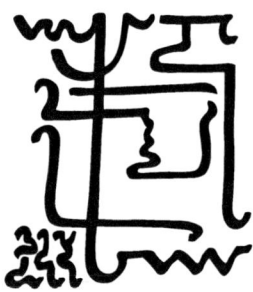

Breath:

- The movement of this slow, steady breath is in the shape of a figure eight with its middle crossover point located behind the navel. The in-breath moves up the left leg, starting from a hand length below the foot. It then crosses over behind the navel to the right side of the body, turning into an out-breath that moves up the right side of the upper torso.
- The out-breath then moves up through the right lung and continues up along the right side of the head. It exits at the top of the right side of the head and moves into the Lahun chakra.
- In the Lahun, the out-breath becomes the in-breath. Drawing the breath in, move it down the left side of the head and upper body to the crossover point behind the navel where it smoothly becomes the out-breath that then moves down the right leg.
- Move the breath out through the bottom of the right foot and into the point, one hand length below the right foot. It then curves across to the same point below the left foot, becoming the in-breath.
- All the gaps between the breaths are eliminated except for the gap between the out-breath and in-breath below the feet.

Eye movements:

- There are no specific eye movements for this posture.

- This cycle consists of 2 breaths. Repeat this pattern of 12 x 2 breaths for a total of 24 breaths.

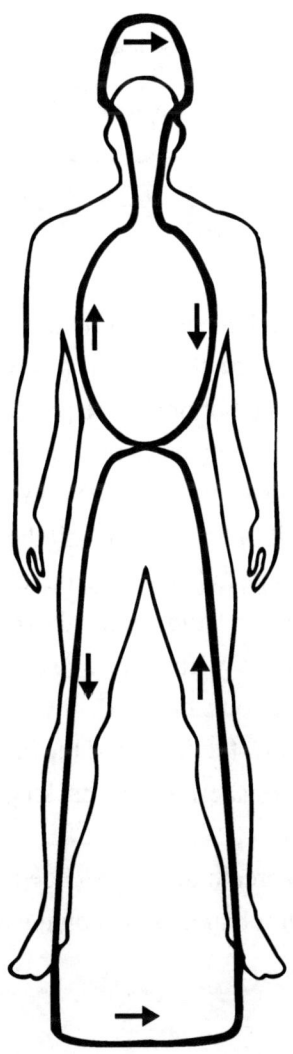

7. *Atma uhu setvrahut ananasvi*
The Breath of the Fountain of Life

I love the totality of my experiences as the revelations of my greater self.

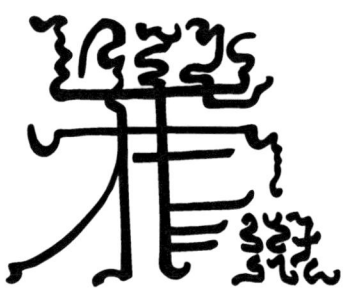

Breath:

- For this final breath, inhale deeply on the in-breath, leaving no gap as you sigh out the out-breath. There is a gap between the out-breath and the in-breath, at the bottom of the pranic tube.
- Pull the breath up the extended pranic tube (it reaches a hand length into the ground as it extends downwards beyond the base of the spine), allowing it to be pulled up all the way into the Lahun chakra. The in-breath goes from the ground all the way to the Lahun chakra, which is a hand length above the crown.
- The in-breath immediately transitions to an out-breath that moves downwards in two arcs outside your body similar to a tube-toral flow. It will move down the front and the back of the body simultaneously, like a waterfall, and back up the extended pranic tube on the in-breath.
- As you repeat the in-breath up the extended pranic tube, this time breathe out in two simultaneous arcs on the outside of your body to the left and right side.

- Alternate the out-breaths by arcing them down the front and back of the body and then on the next out-breath, down both sides of the body.

Eye movements:
- There are no specific eye movements for this breath.

- Repeat the exercise for 12 cycles of in- and out-breaths.
- After you have completed the 12 breaths, rest and allow time for contemplation on the following principle:

> *Death and life are two simultaneous aspects of my eternal being. They express inseparably through my endless and beginningless existence.*

Note: At death, the being's soul leaves through the crown. In life, only the pranic tube within the body (from the base of the spine to the crown) is used. During the being's time in the soul world of the dead, only the pranic tube from the base of the spine to a hand length into the ground is used. During life in the uterus, the soul moves through the base of the spine, into the upper part of the pranic tube within the body. By using the full pranic tube, as done in the 7th breath, immortality can be achieved.

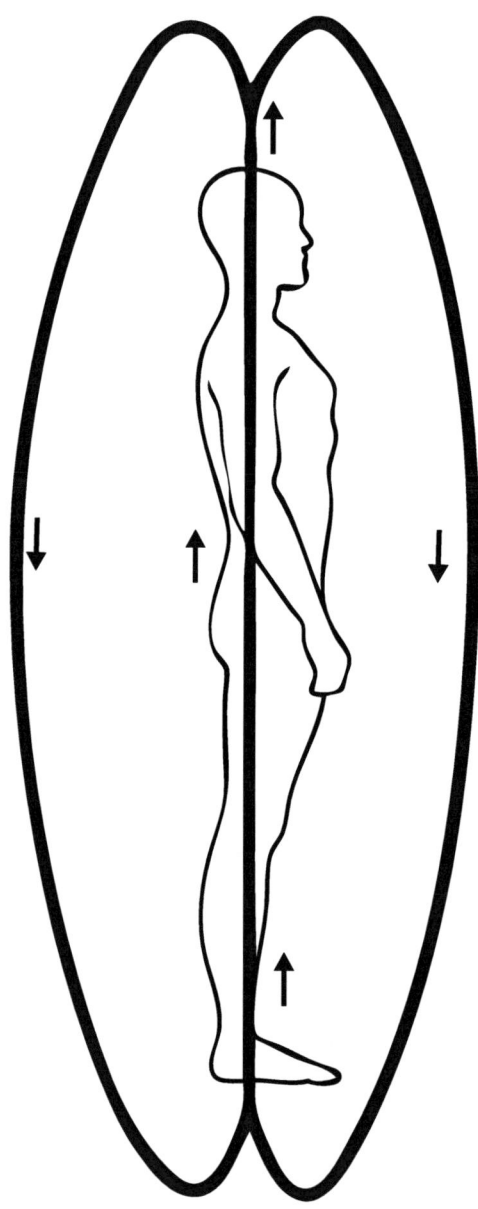

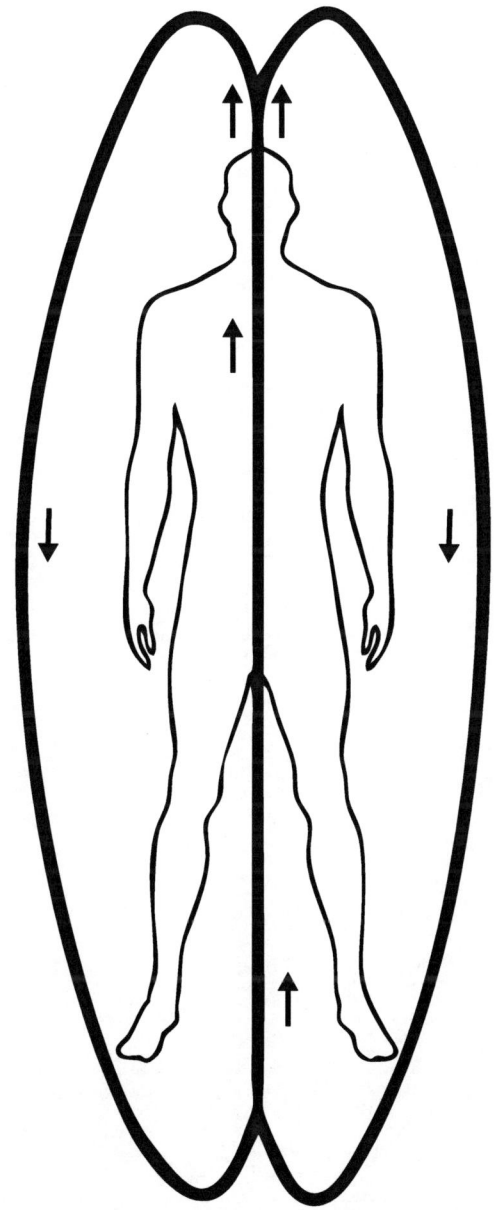

The Arasatma Breaths Level II

Activating Self-regeneration of Resources

*The body's ability to rest within activity
becomes activated when our being becomes
our sustenance. The peace of eternal life
floods our being.*

Paintings for Level II Arasatma Breaths

Almine has created a specific painting for each breath in Level II that can be meditated upon prior to doing each breath. They embody the principles of each breath, depict their colors and train the eyes to see beyond the illusion of solidity and static, fossilized form. These paintings are available as an addition to the Level II breathing techniques. For details on how you can purchase them see the front of this book.

If using the paintings for meditation, observe their fluid lines and how one area flows into another. Realize that your life flows just like the paintings.

Having purchased these paintings you may then want to place them in your environment as a reminder of the fluidness of life.

Guidelines for Level II

It is recommended that Level I be practiced at for at least five days before moving on to Level II.

Once again, the first 4 breaths are done in a seated position with the spine straight and legs crossed. The remaining 3 breaths are done while lying down.

As you do the exercises, play the musical elixir that has been specifically created to accompany the Arasatma Breaths.

In Level II hand mudras (positions) are incorporated, as well as the envisioning of the breaths as colors. Where eye movements are included, these may be done with either your eyes closed or open, as preferred.

For each of the exercises, the breaths should be repeated 12 times (the in- and out-breath count as one breath), except for Breath 6 which consists of 2 breaths for each cycle, making a total of 24 breaths.

When breathing for these exercises, draw the breath in (inhale) through the nose and blow the breath out (exhale) through the mouth.

For breaths 1 – 6, the breath circles within the body. Breath 7 circles outside the body.

You may wish to place the sigils that accompany these breaths in front of you to look at during the exercises.

These techniques facilitate the release of bodily toxins, so it is advisable that you increase your intake of water. You may also experience some heat and the release of emotions, as well as the appearance of images from your past either during the breaths or after them.

1. Atma seba uhut
The Breath of the Lion's Gate

I acknowledge that my reality is a fluid expression of Infinite Intent. The seeming static nature of matter is due to the limited capacities of the senses.

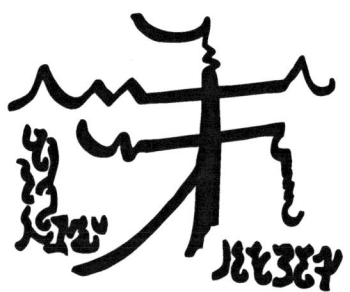

Hand mudra:

- While sitting with your spine straight and your legs crossed, take the tips of the middle fingers and touch the tips of the thumbs of each hand. Rest your hands, palms up, on your knees.

Eye movements:

- As you breathe in and out, your eyes will move to match the in- and out-breaths. Start with your eyes looking down towards the ground and as you breathe in, slowly raise your eyes up towards the sky. As you breathe out, slowly lower your eyes down again. Repeat with each breath.

Colors:

- Envision the breath as a violet flow of intense color as you move it in its circuit.

Tongue:
- Push the tip of the tongue into the roof of the mouth (at the front of the hard palate).

The Breath:
- The in-breath will cycle from the atlas joint (the place where the skull and the neck meet), up the back of the skull, out of the crown and into the Lahun chakra.
- The out-breath will cycle down from the Lahun chakra, around the front of the skull, down the face and back to the atlas joint at the back of the neck.
- Both the in- and out-breaths circle inside the skull. The duration of each in- and out-breath is for about the count of 5.
- Repeat for 12 cycles of in- and out-breaths.

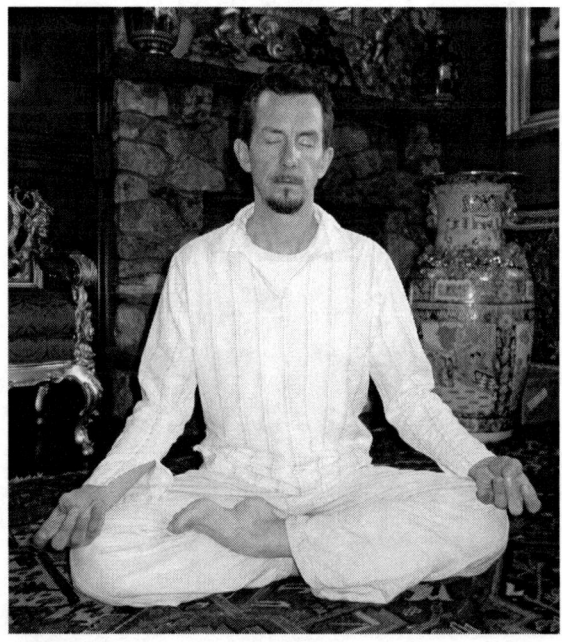

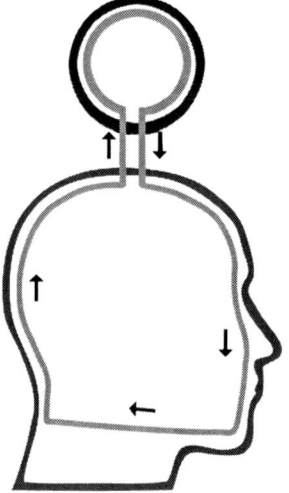

2. *Atma avi uhet nanastu*
The Breath of the Winged Ones

In sleep I have wakefulness, when awake I am resting.
Through surrendered trust, I am in passive receptivity
during proactivity.

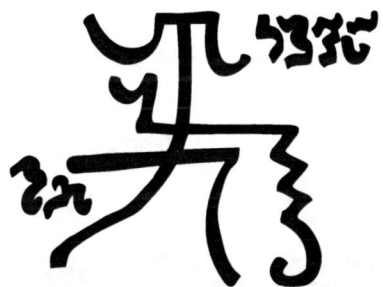

The Hand Mudra:
- With interlocking fingers and palms up, place your hands upon your diaphragm; rest the hands lightly against your body to allow for movement of the chest from side to side.

The Colors:
- The breath when drawn into the left lung is turquoise.
- When you fill the right lung, the breath is emerald green.
- The breaths will alternate between these two colors with the in-breath on the left side being turquoise and the in-breath on the right side being emerald green.

Eye movements:
- For this exercise in Level II, eye movements are incorporated along with the breathing. As you breathe, move the eyes left as you fill the left lung. Move the eyes slowly to the right as you exhale. The eyes will be all the way to the right when you fill the right lung and move to the left as you breathe out and move the ribs to the left. In summary, the eyes follow the movements of the chest.

39

The Breath:

- Inhaling deeply, move the rib cage to the left. Keep the rest of the torso and head as still as possible.
- As you breathe out slowly, move the rib cage to the right. When you have moved the rib cage to the right, pause and inhale deeply into the right lung. As you slowly exhale, move the rib cage to the left.
- Pause, inhale deeply into the left lung and then move the rib cage to the right again.
- Repeat for 12 cycles of in- and out-breaths.

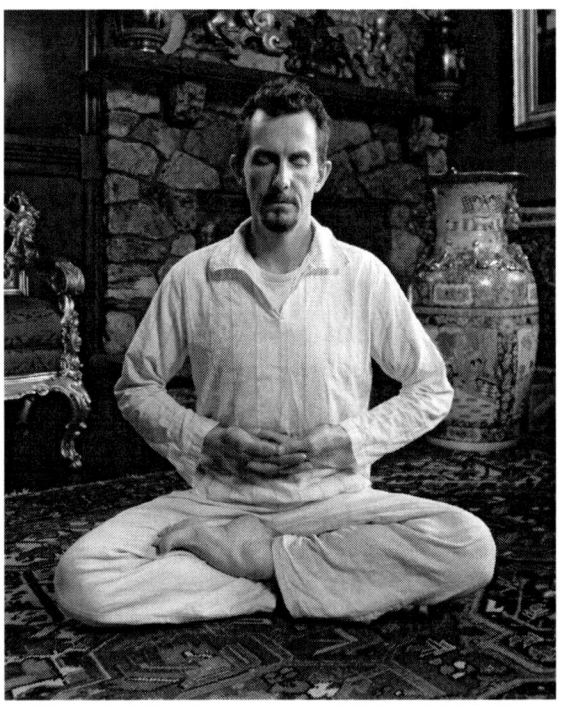

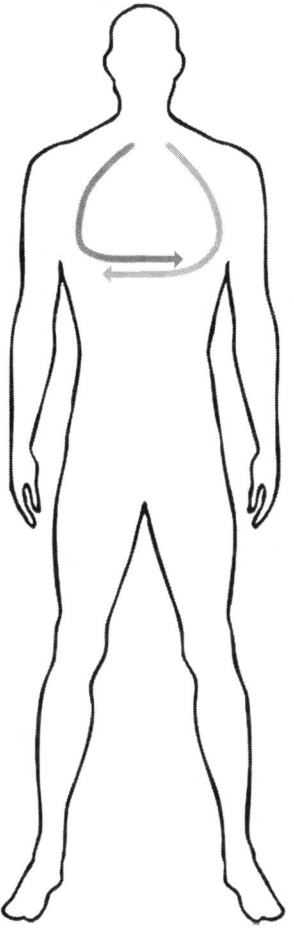

*Pause before inhaling deeply into the left lung, visualizing the
breath as turquoise. Then, move the rib cage to the right as
you exhale, breathing out the turquoise breath.*

*Pause before inhaling deeply into the right lung, visualizing
the breath as emerald green. Then, move the rib cage to the
left as you exhale, breathing out the emerald green breath.*

3. *Krihet atma unanes tuvi*
The Breath of Heaven and Earth

I release all that I hold onto and cut any cords of control.

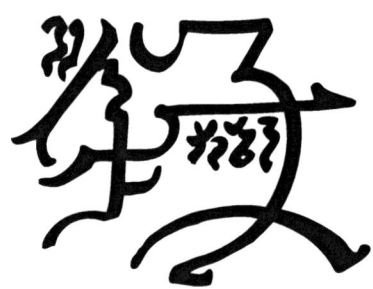

Hand Mudra:
- Interlock the fingers of both hands and with palms up; place them right above the pubic bone. Hold them in this position throughout Breath 3.

Colors:
- The breath is envisioned as a yellow current of air swirling around the abdomen. It is bright yellow on the inhale and becomes a beautiful clear amber as you exhale.

Eye movements:
- The eyes match the rotation of the breath. Start by looking down as you breathe in and then rotate your eyes to the right and up as you finish the in-breath. As you breathe out, rotate your eyes to the left and then downward as you complete the out-breath at the pubic bone.

The Breath:
- Starting at the midpoint directly above the pubic bone, breathe in deeply, moving the breath in a circular pattern up the right side of the body to the top of the abdomen (where the diaphragm is located).
- The breath is slowly blown out as it circles down the left side of the abdomen back to the the midpoint above the pubic bone.
- Repeat for 12 cycles of in- and out-breaths.

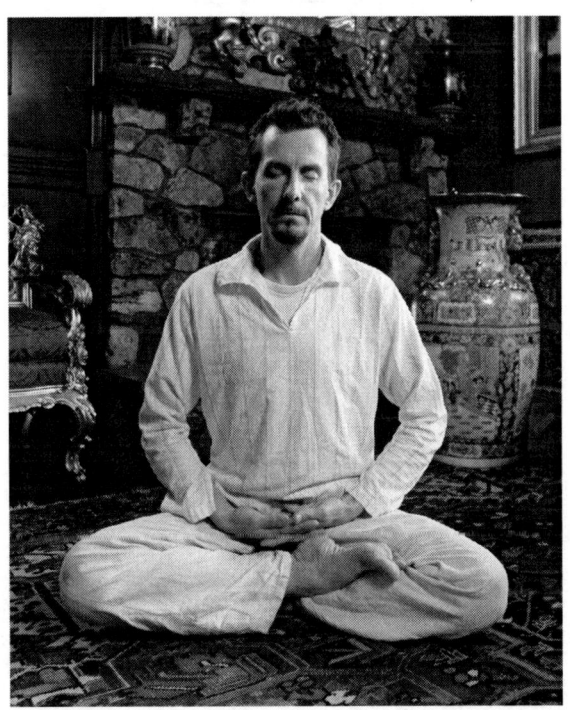

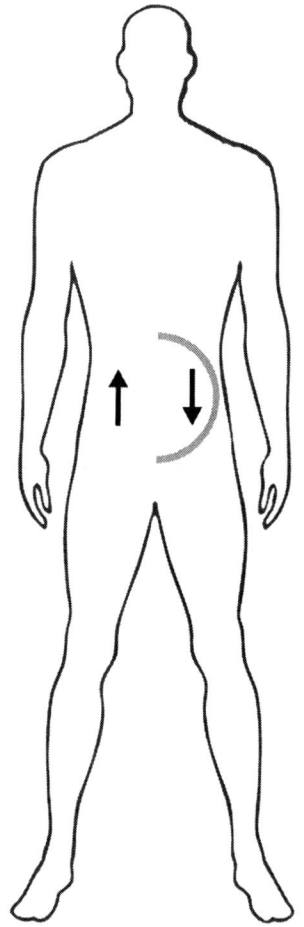

The Wheel for Opening the Navel Area and the Purification of the Life Force Center

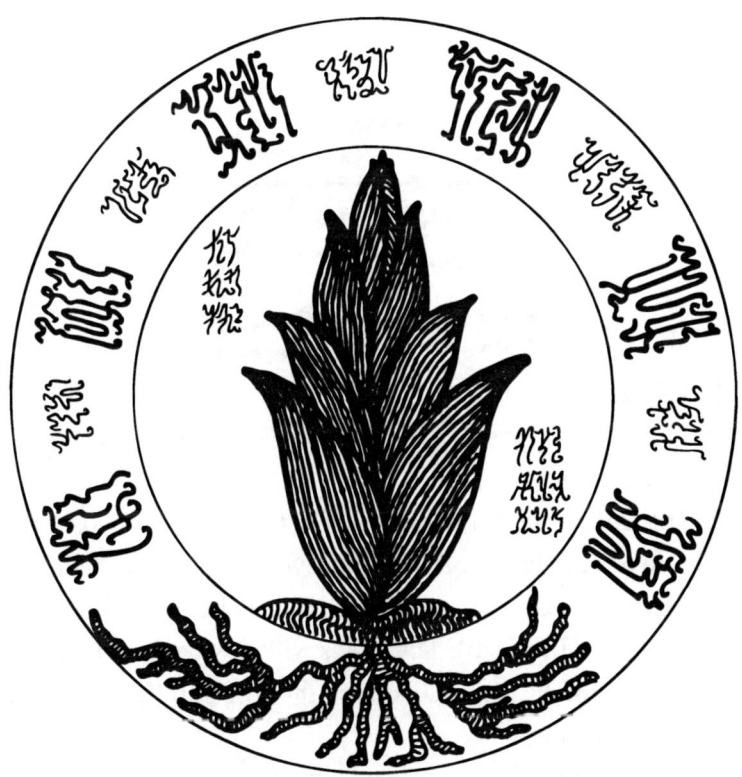

Kaarech Mishavet Eresta Uvasvi

4. *Atma utu kranavesvi uhut*
The Breath of the Little Horn

I am the sovereign creator of my own reality. The ability to affect the quality of my journey, begins with accepting full responsibility for the way in which Infinite Intent expresses through me.

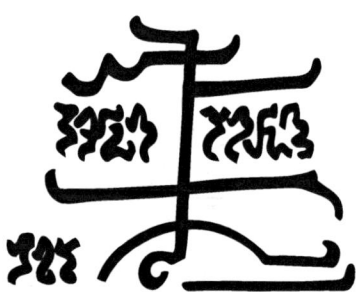

Hand Mudra:

- To find the correct position of the hands, begin by placing the tips of the middle fingers of both hands together. Then place the tips of your thumbs together to create a circle with your hands. Place the circle of your hands around the navel, resting them lightly on the abdomen. Then, keeping the hands in a circle, move the fingers 5 inches apart (12-13cm). The hands will now be forming a larger circle in the middle of the abdomen (they are still lightly resting on the stomach area).
- The position of the hands indicate where the breath will build prior to being forced down the lower pranic tube. Maintain the hand position during the breath.

Colors:

- As you draw the breath in through the top of your head down the pranic tube, it is brilliant white. As it builds in the navel area, it becomes a vivid electric blue (slightly darker than the sky) and changes to an intense blue on the out-breath.

Eye movements:
- Eyes remain looking forward for this breath.

The Breath:
- Draw the breath in from the top of the head and down to the navel. Inhale as deeply as possible.
- Forcefully expel the breath down from the navel and out the base of the spine, blowing out all debris of the past and straightening the pranic tube.
- Repeat for 12 cycles of in- and out-breaths.

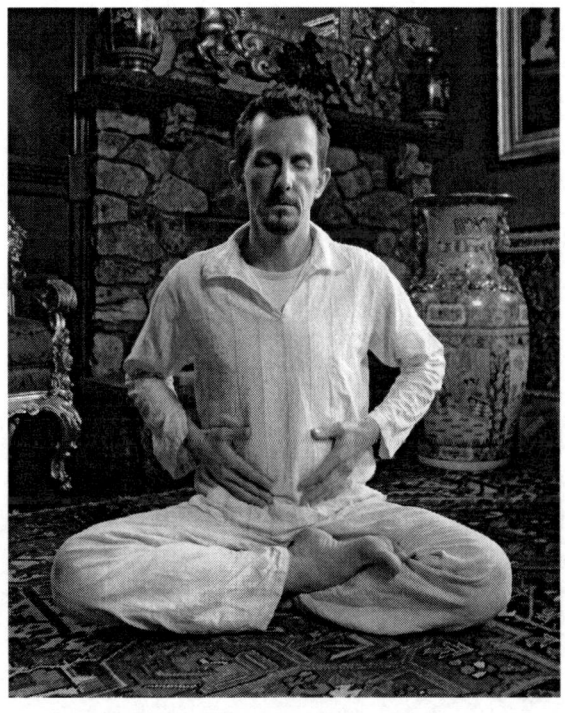

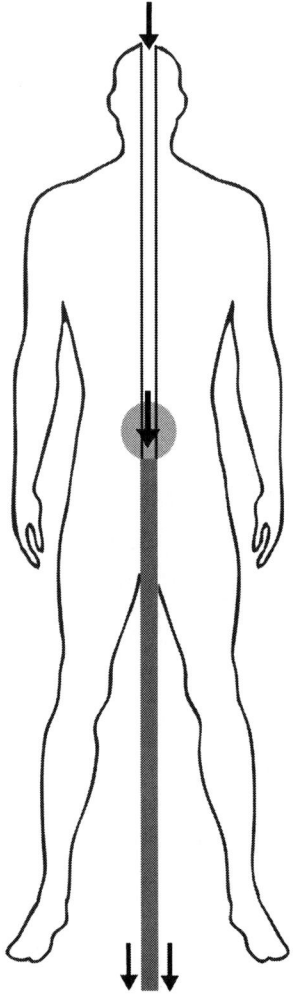

5. *Selva nechtasu atma karanu*
The Breath of the Fire Walk

*There is neither success nor failure upon the innocent
journey of self-discovery. In the freedom of this knowledge,
I explore life's revelations.*

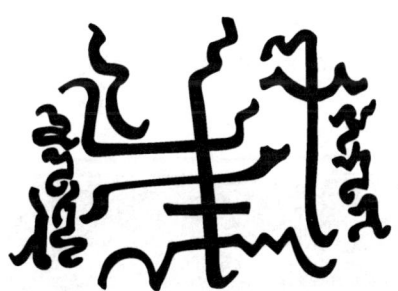

Hand Mudra:
- As the breath is pulled up the left leg, tap the side of the left hand (between the bottom of the small finger and the wrist) with two fingers from the right hand. In many people this is the fleshy part of the hand.
- As you breathe out down the right leg, tap the same spot on the right hand with two fingers from the left hand.

Colors:
- As you inhale, envision the breath as the color orange. As it arcs across the abdomen, becoming the out-breath, the color changes to red. Continue envisioning these two colors for each of the breaths.

The Breath:
- Lying down with your legs straight, draw the in-breath up the left leg, from a point one hand length below the left foot. As the breath moves up the left leg and continues into the lower abdomen, it arcs across to the right hip.

- Breathe out, moving the breath down the right leg and into a point one hand length below the right foot.
- As it arcs across to the same point below the left foot, the out-breath becomes the in-breath.
- There are no gaps either between the in-breath and the out-breath, or between the out-breath and the in-breath. The transition between all breaths must be smooth.
- Repeat for 12 cycles of in- and out-breaths.

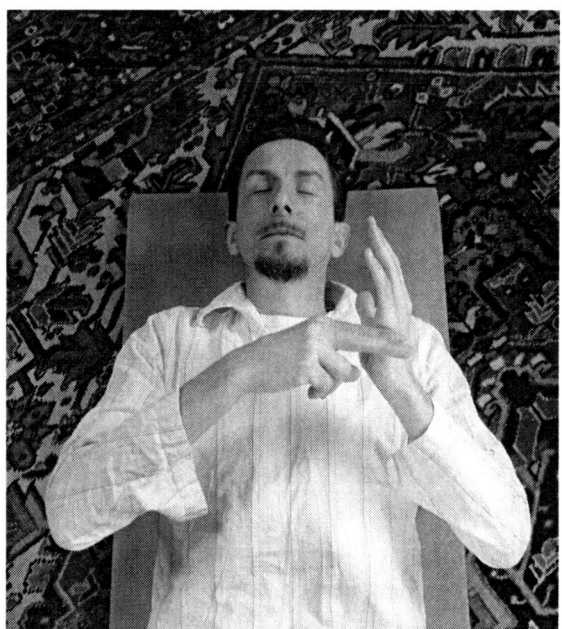

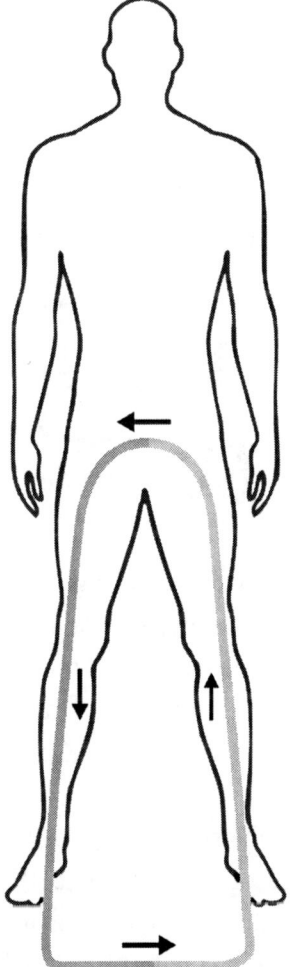

6. *Atma usu amara-uhet*
The Breath of the Divine Marriage

Humility is not based on comparison, one thing being less than another, but by acknowledging the unknowableness of existence. True humility is the foundation of mastery.

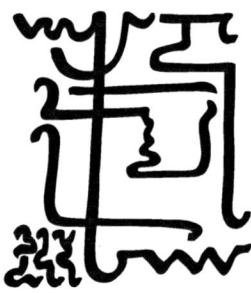

Hand Mudra:

- As you lie down, your hands are lying in a relaxed position next to your body, with the thumb and middle finger of the left hand touching tip to tip and the thumb and middle finger of the right hand touching tip to tip. The palms are facing up.

The Colors:

- The key to unlocking the second level of power of this breath is in the visualization of color as you breathe. Begin by seeing a pulsing bright yellow light around the navel, about the size of a grapefruit.
- As you draw the breath up the left leg, it will be orange. As it moves through the yellow ball of light at the navel to become the out-breath and moves up the right side of the body, it turns emerald green.
- At the Lahun chakra, the out-breath becomes the in-breath, and is turquoise as it moves down the left side of the upper body. As it moves through the yellow ball at the navel, it becomes magenta on

the out-breath. Exhale the magenta all the way down the right leg and into the ground, a hand length below the right foot.

- The breath then becomes orange again as it arcs across to the same point below the left foot and continues up the left leg.

The Breath:

- The movement of this breath is in the shape of a figure eight with its middle crossover point located behind the navel. There are no gaps between the breaths, transitioning smoothly from the in-breath to the out-breath and visa versa.
- The in-breath moves up the left leg, starting from a hand length below the foot. It then crosses over to the right, behind the navel, and turns into an out-breath that moves up the right side of the upper torso.
- The out-breath them moves up through the right lung and continues up along the right side of the face. It exits at the top of the head and moves into the Lahun chakra.
- In the Lahun, the out-breath becomes the in-breath. Drawing the breath in, move it down the left side of the head and upper body to the crossover point behind the navel, where it smoothly becomes the out-breath that moves down the right leg.
- Move the breath out through the bottom of the right foot and into a point, one hand length below the right foot. It then curves across to the same point below the left foot, becoming the in-breath.
- The full figure eight consisting of 2 full in- and out-breaths, must be repeated 12 times (24 breaths in total).

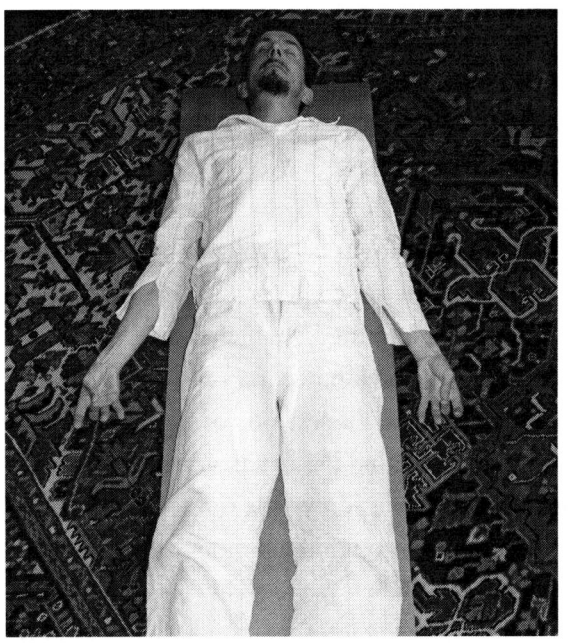

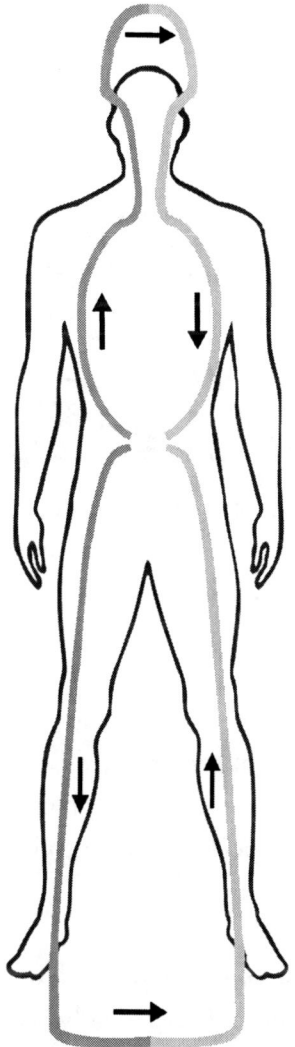

7. *Atma uhu setvrahut ananasvi*
The Breath of the Fountain of Life.

I have become the Fountain of Life. Every creature in my environment flourishes as I express the fullness of my being.

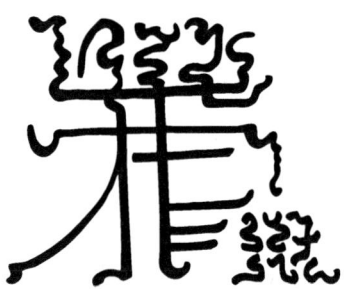

Up to this point, the previous 6 breaths have created integrated harmony of body and soul. This final breath creates harmonious interaction of the body, soul and spirit.

Hand Mudra:

• Lying on your back, bring the fingertips of the left hand to touch the fingertips of the right hand and rest your hands lightly over the heart area. The fingers may either point towards your chin or towards the ceiling, depending on which is most comfortable.

The Colors:

• As the breath is drawn up the full length of the pranic tube, it will start out as a vivid blue color, gradually becoming lighter until it is a brilliant white as it reaches the navel. It stays white all the way into the Lahun chakra. As it bursts into the out-breath, it becomes bright golden yellow, moving as a full tube torus in all directions until it becomes blue on the in-breath again.

The Breath:

- For this final breath, breathe deeply on the in-breath and sigh it out on the out-breath with no gap between the in-breath and the out-breath. The gap between the out-breath and the in-breath below the feet is maintained.
- As you inhale deeply, draw the breath up the extended pranic tube, from a hand length into the ground, all the way up to the Lahun chakra, above the crown.
- The in-breath immediately transitions to an out-breath that moves outwards and downwards in a full 360° arc outside and around the body. The arc will be a full tube torus, rolling outward in trillions of golden yellow fibers reaching all the way into the ground and then becomes the in-breath as it travels back up the extended pranic tube.
- Repeat for 12 cycles of in- and out-breaths.
- After the 12 repetitions are completed, allow time to lie in stillness without any thought.

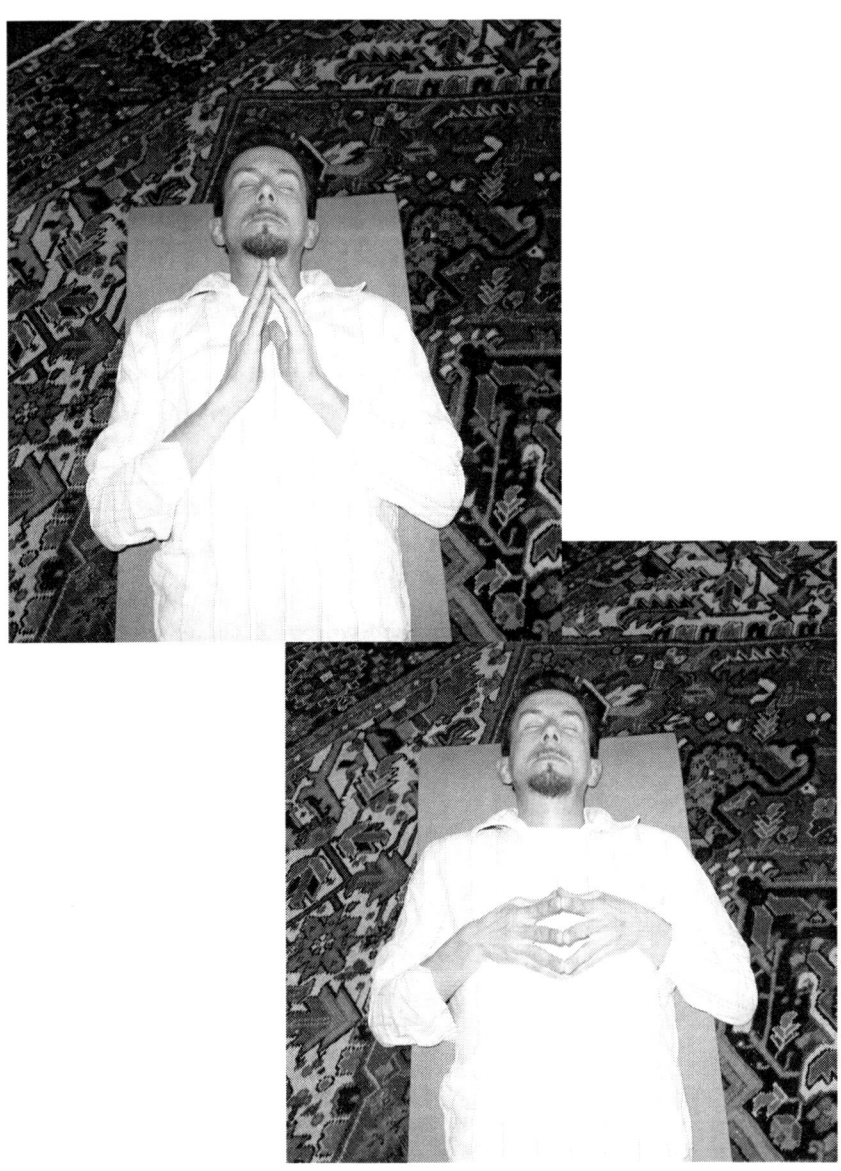

Choose whichever hand position is most comfortable.

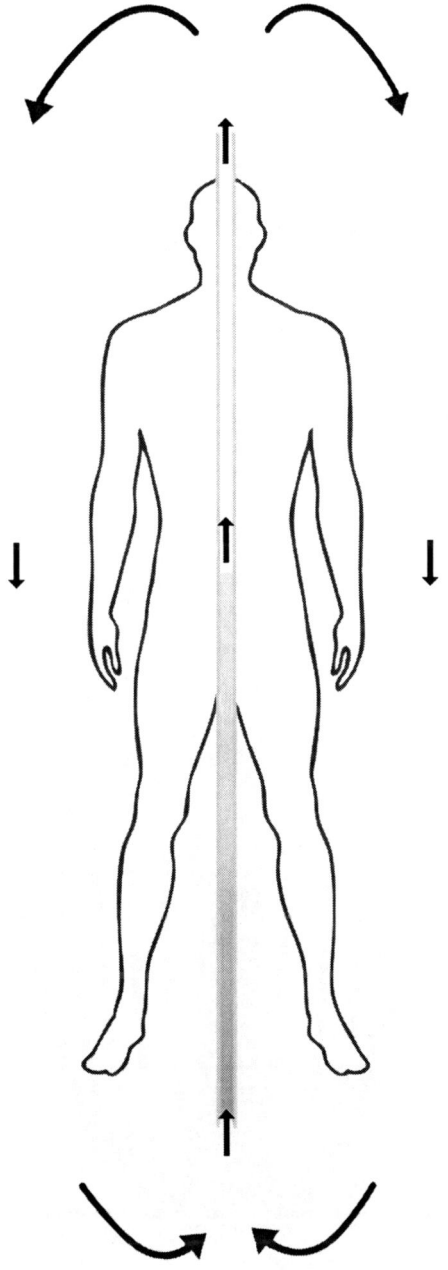

The Arasatma Breaths Level III

Evolving the DNA into Higher Expression

*The origin of war comes from the separation
of the DNA strands. Being opposites of
one another, they are in an antagonistic
relationship.*

Introduction to Level III

The primary origin of shame comes from the cosmic ascent into light during half of its cycles around the massive cosmic orbit. During the light ascension, frequency descends or grows less. During this time perception peaks but emotions are more flat and unfeeling. From a heightened perception state, looking back at past choices, it is inconceivable to imagine that we made such poor decisions. This produces shame and guilt.

As emotions grow less during a light ascension, we can act in an unfeeling way towards others. This creates emotional karma and deep regrets, especially when we look at the past from the height of the ascension of frequency – a time when emotions run high. Emotional karma is resolved after death. The emotional karma makes humanity subject to death, and the karma of deeds resulting from 'wrong' choices, pulls us back into rebirth.

The 300 positions of the cosmos, as it rotates around its orbit, have 150 positions of ascending light (descending in frequency). The other side of the orbit has 150 positions of ascending frequency (descending in light). Since these fluctuations in perception and frequency (emotion) are the cause of karma, this in turn causes life and death, and true freedom lies in overcoming them. The macrocosmic phenomenon is mirrored in man, the microcosm. At the apex of his evolution, the god-kingdom, he functions from 300 strands of DNA. In overcoming these cycles, all 300 DNA strands function as one, with alternating emphasis as required.

The DNA has to evolve from two twisted strands of 150 strands each (resembling a figure 8), to a single untwisted cord of 300 strands functioning as one. The figure 8 has to become a cooperative circle – the two twisted ropes of DNA are separate and create the origin of war.

The complete overcoming of value judgments and the release of regrets is the major component of this dramatic evolution of the DNA.

Breath is a valuable tool for changing not only the attitudes of judgementalism but the DNA itself. The third level of the Arasatma breaths accomplishes this.

The Positions of the Cosmos During the Ascension and Descension Cycles

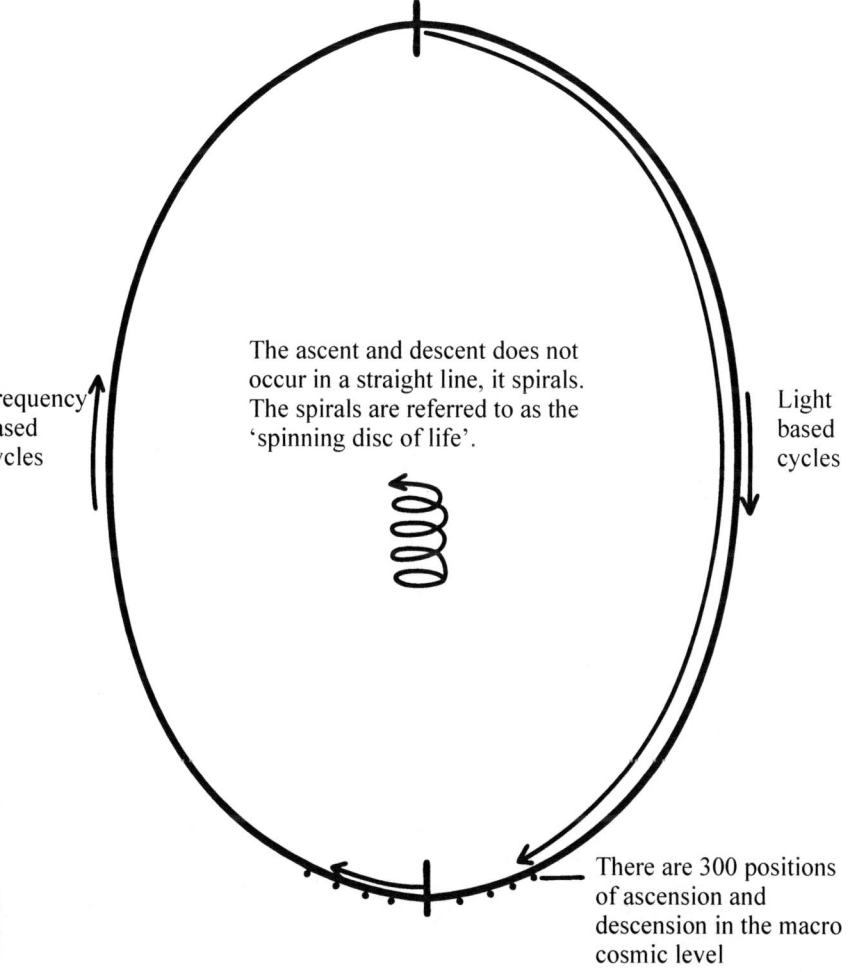

Frequency based cycles

Light based cycles

The ascent and descent does not occur in a straight line, it spirals. The spirals are referred to as the 'spinning disc of life'.

There are 300 positions of ascension and descension in the macro cosmic level

Guidelines for Level III

It is recommended that Level II be practiced for at least 5 days before moving on to Level III.

In Level III, hand mudras (positions) are also incorporated. The breaths of Level III have no specific colors but colors will light up in the inner space of your being.

Breaths 1 – 4 are done in a sitting position with the spine straight and legs crossed. Breaths 5 – 7 are done lying down.

The sound elixirs that accompany the Arasatma Breaths are used for Level III. Listen to the music as you do the breaths. The elixirs work in conjunction with the breaths, using the alchemical potencies of frequency incorporated within them.

When breathing for these exercises, draw the breath in (inhale) through the nose and blow the breath out (exhale) through the mouth.

There are 12 cycles of in- and out-breaths for each exercise. However, having completed the 12th breath for exercise 7, you may continue with further breaths as you experience the combining of inner and outer space.

As these techniques facilitate the release of bodily toxins, it is advised that you increase your intake of water.

1. *Atma seba uhut*
The Breath of the Lion's Gate

*Through trusting surrender, the grand adventure of my
existence inspires me into fuller expression.*

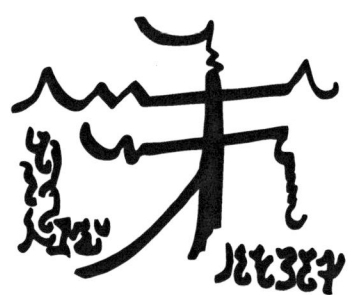

Hand mudra:
- While sitting in a cross-legged position, with your head and spine straight, place the tip of the index finger of your left hand on the left side of your head, about one inch from the outer corner of the eye. (One inch is about the length of the top digit of your middle finger.) This point is the soft part of the temple.
- Place the tip of the index finger of your right hand on the similar point on the right side of your head. Maintain a firm but comfortable pressure on these points during the 12 repetitions of this breath.

The Breath:
- Fill your head with the in-breath. Holding the breath for as long as you can, see the space inside of the head light up with white light and as you hold it, colors may appear.
- Breathe out as slowly as you can, seeing the white light and colors grow dimmer but not disappear. Build the display of colors like a growing work of art with each in-breath. As you move to the next breath, be aware that the illuminated parts of your inner space remain lit and dynamically expressing.

- Repeat for 12 cycles of in- and out-breaths.

Points on the Temple

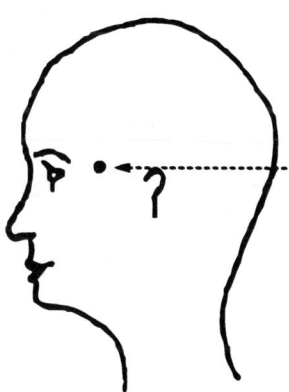

Note: The ancient Egyptian culture used to extend the eye make-up they wore to these points on the temples. This was to mark the position of the points of the Aubari – the source of clairaudience.

2. *Atma avi uhet nanastu*
The Breath of the Winged Ones

Through appreciative awareness, the unfolding perception and beauty of my eternal being reveals itself to me.

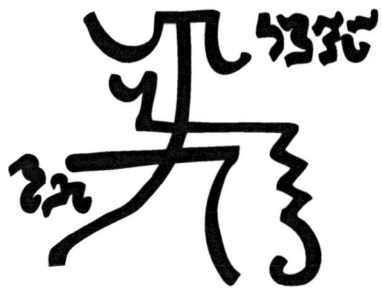

Hand Mudra:

- For the second breath, remain in a cross-legged position with your spine and head straight. Place your hands, with finger tips about one hand length apart and palms facing upwards, just below your ribcage and above your abdomen.

The Breath:

- Inhale deeply, filling the lungs and chest cavity with as much air as possible. Hold the breath for as long as you can.
- See the lungs and chest cavity fill with white light. The heart will pulsate red, orange and on through all the colors of the rainbow. With each pulsation, the light within the chest cavity grows brighter.
- Breathe out as slowly as you can. The chest will remain lit but becomes dimmer during the out-breath.
- Repeat for 12 cycles of in- and out-breaths.

3. *Krihet atma unanes tuvi*
The Breath of Heaven and Earth

*I dwell in ever-renewed wonderment and rapture at the
majesty of infinite life in finite expression.*

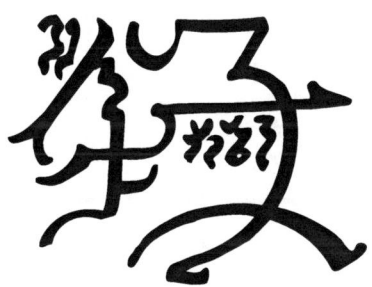

Hand Mudra:

- In a cross-legged, seated position, rest your hands on your thighs.
  The hands are relaxed with palms facing upwards and thumbs and
  index fingers touching. Keep the thumbs and index fingers together
  with a steady pressure throughout the 12 repetitions of this breath.

The Breath:

- Inhaling deeply, fill the abdomen with as much breath as possible.
  Make a point of distending the stomach on the in-breath. The
  stomach should move out as far as possible during the in-breath,
  falling back to its original position on the out-breath.
- Holding the in-breath for as long as possible, see the abdomen
  fill with scene after scene of field flowers, song birds, clean rivers
  full of fish, thriving animal life and scenes of fulfilled and happy
  people living in harmony with the Earth. Create an inspirational
  scene for each of the 12 breaths, similar to the those that are
  described above.
- As you exhale a long, slow out-breath, the scenes you chose to
  envision move from your inner space to the outer surroundings of

your life. Know that as you breathe out, somewhere on Earth, it becomes an actual reality.

- Repeat for 12 cycles of in- and out-breaths.

4. *Atma utu kranavesvi uhut*
The Breath of the Little Horn

I observe myself as the many, through omniperspective
perception rooted in inner vision.

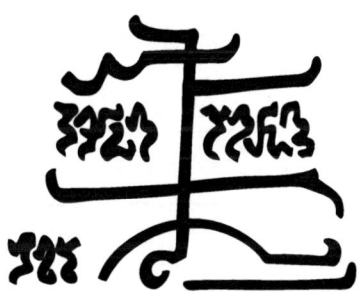

Hand Mudra:
- In a seated position, your hands are resting palms up on your thighs, thumbs and middle fingers touching.

The Breath:
- Breathe in deeply and hold the breath for as long as possible while envisioning something that stirs positive feelings in your heart (such as feelings of tenderness when seeing the innocence of a newly hatched chick you hold in your hands). Each of the 12 repetitions of this breath will have a unique and different envisioned scene and resulting feeling.
- Fill your whole torso, chest, neck and head with the in-breath. Breathing in, the color is bright white but as you exhale the color will change. Do not pay attention to the colors as they change on the out-breath.
- As you exhale, breathe out through the base of the spine. The out-breath will be long and deep as you allow the specific positive feelings felt on the in-breath to flow into the Earth. See them spread throughout the form of the planet, like a colored wind.

- The depth to which you can experience the positive feelings, while holding the in-breath, is very important. To find the depth of these feelings, draw from the things that you love and from happy memories of touching moments. Keep the feelings as the focus of your awareness as you breathe them throughout the Earth.

- Repeat for 12 cycles of in- and out-breaths.

5. *Selva nechtasu atma karanu*
The Breath of the Fire Walk

Through the eternal perspective of omnisensory vision, the
harmlessness of the timeless journey is revealed.

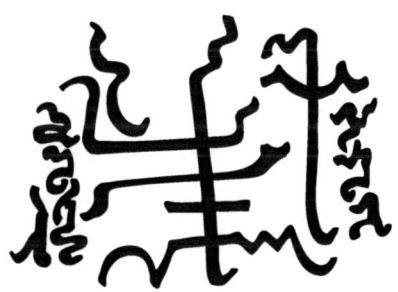

Hand Mudra:
- Lie flat on your back, with your arms relaxed by your sides, palms facing upwards.

The Breath:
- The 12 repetitions of this breath are progressive in that they build on one another, culminating in magnitude during the 12th in-breath.
- Breathe in deeply while imagining your body growing larger and larger. See your body as a field rather than a solid mass, easily able to expand with each in-breath. Fill the expanding field with white light.
- As you gently relax and breathe out, see the expanded field stay as enlarged as it was on the previous in-breath. Build the field larger and larger with each in-breath. Start by building it as large as the whole Earth. The next inhale would build it to the size of solar system, then the galaxy, until eventually it is the size of the cosmos. The in-breaths are emphasized over the out-breaths.

- Repeat for 12 cycles of in- and out-breaths.
- On the last out-breath contemplate the following:

Chevech huras estavi mananech stuhabit ukleshvi haruset prihabat kluvaveshvi arsanat. Kreha uvanat sebahut arsanach ubli vrihurasatvi ananes.

All I can ever experience or perceive is created by that which I emphasize or suppress. I am the sovereign cause of my reality.

6. *Atma usu amara-uhet*
The Breath of the Divine Marriage

I exist in inspired illumination, expressing as a living work of art.

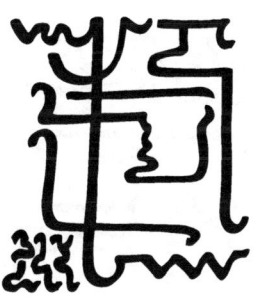

Hand Mudra:

- Remain in the same position, lying flat with your arms and hands lying in a relaxed position by your side, palms up. Know yourself to be a being as vast as the cosmos having a human experience.

The Breath:

- Inhale as deeply and powerfully as you can. As you do, fill the entire cosmos with a diaphanous and transparent white light. Feel your awareness expand across planets, suns and galaxies during the in-breath.
- As you breathe out, contract back to the body, again sweeping your awareness over the cosmic space.
- Repeat 12 times, allowing the in- and out-breaths to be like a massive cosmic pulse.
- On the last out-breath contemplate the following:

Michba rutvi aharanasvava ukret piravit erchta vri uhurunasba.
I effect all through the passion and joy of my existence.

7. *Atma uhu setvrahut ananasvi*
The Breath of the Fountain of Life

I appreciate the poetry of the dance of light and shadow without judgement.

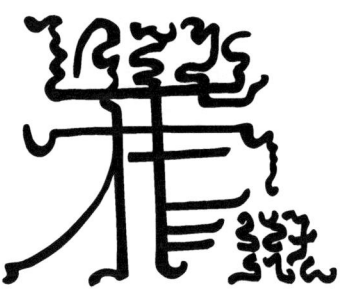

Note: The in- and out-breath in the outer space around you and the in- and out-breath of your inner space (in other words breaths 1 – 11) count as one breath.

Hand Mudra:
- Lying flat, make a circle with your hands by placing your middle fingers tip to tip and the thumbs of both hands tip to tip. Place this circle, palms down, around your belly button. See your navel as the bridge between your inner space and the space without.

The Breath:
- The first 11 in- and out-breaths are similar. The 12th breath of this exercise is different; it is the culmination of the previous 11 breaths.
- There is a pause between the in-breath and the out-breath with every out-breath being similar to a rapid collapse (like letting a stretched elastic band go). There is no gap between the out-breath and the in-breath.

- As you inhale the first breath, breathe in deeply, filling the entire cosmos around you with your presence as a form of transparent luminosity.
- Pause before you exhale and feel the fullness of your presence and expression. As you exhale (like a rapid collapse), contract your awareness to the belly button.
- Inhale without any pause, filling your inner cosmos/universe with your presence. Prior to exhaling, pause to feel the fullness of your inner presence and expression. As you exhale, contract your inner vision back to the navel and without a pause, inhale.
- As you breathe in again, fill the outer cosmos with breath. In this way, alternate between the outer and inner space for the first 11 breaths, using the navel as a doorway between them.
- For the 12th in-breath, breathe deeply into your inner cosmic space, filling it with your breath. As you transition to the out-breath, forcefully expel the breath with the intent of bursting the imaginary boundary between inner and outer space. The movement of the breath is similar to the folding movement of the tube torus. The breath moves to the edge of the tube torus on the in-breath and folds over and back to the center on the out-breath.
- On bursting the boundary between inner and outer space you will discover that they have always been one.
- As you feel the after effects of combining inner and outer space, you may want to continue with more rotational breaths. Only the 12th breath uses forceful expulsion on the out-breath. After that, the breaths flow in a smooth circle, in and out. Do as many breaths, after breath 12, as you wish.

Contemplate the following:

I am the boundless ocean. No division can exist within my being.

Breath 7 - The Fountain of Life
The Movement of the First 11 Breaths

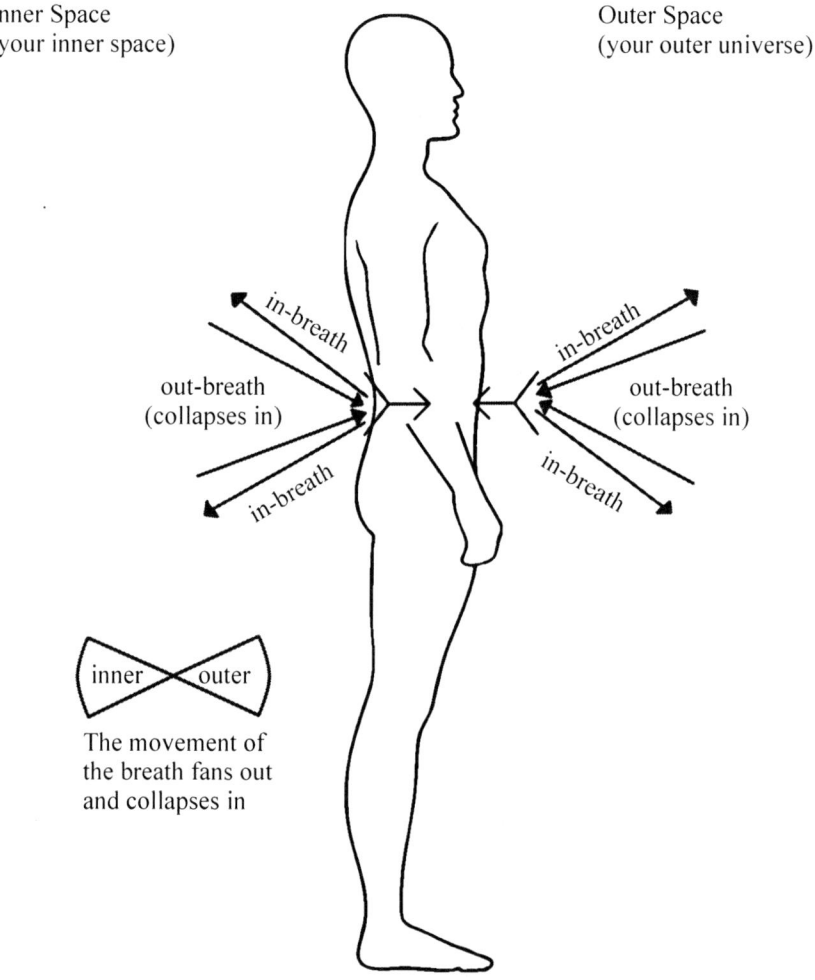

Inner Space
(your inner space)

Outer Space
(your outer universe)

in-breath

in-breath

out-breath
(collapses in)

out-breath
(collapses in)

in-breath

in-breath

inner ✕ outer

The movement of
the breath fans out
and collapses in

The Movement of the 12th Breath

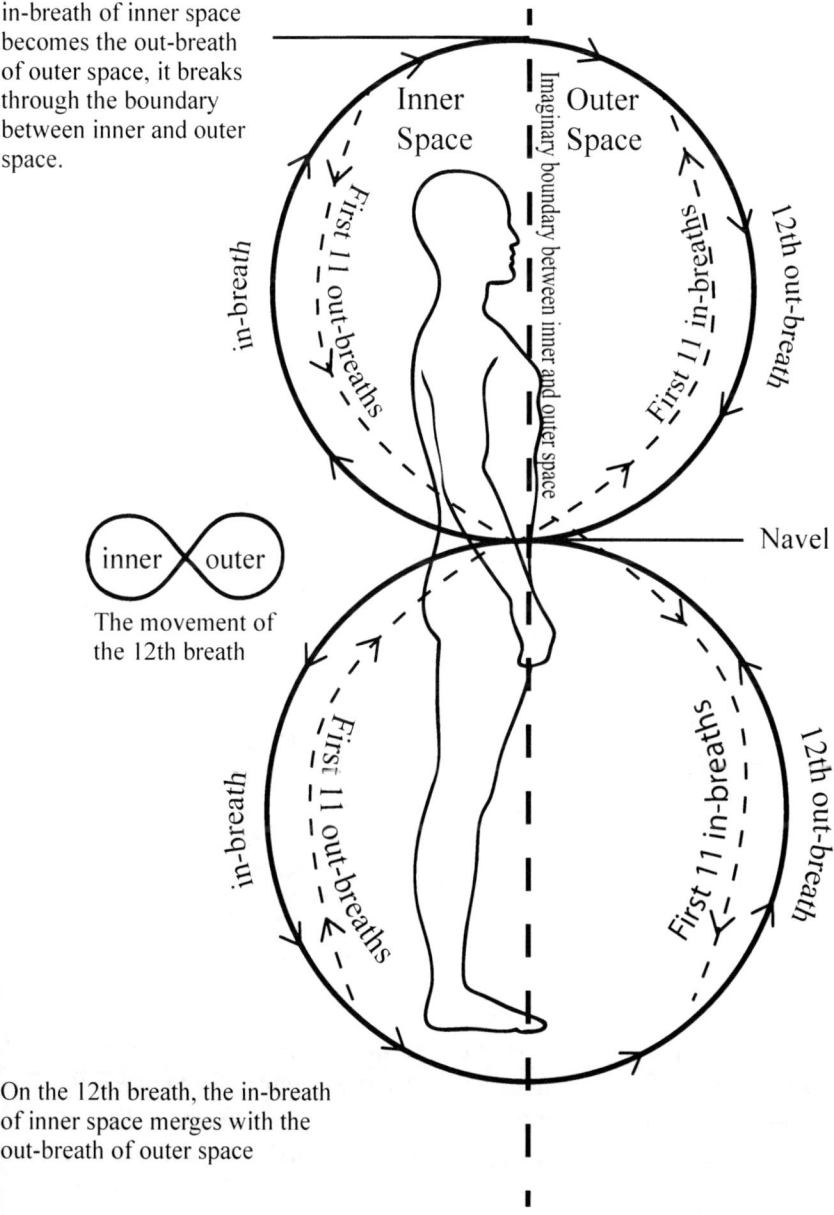

On the 12th breath, as the in-breath of inner space becomes the out-breath of outer space, it breaks through the boundary between inner and outer space.

Inner Space

Outer Space

Imaginary boundary between inner and outer space

in-breath

First 11 out-breaths

First 11 in-breaths

12th out-breath

inner ⟋⟍ outer

The movement of the 12th breath

Navel

First 11 out-breaths

in-breath

First 11 in-breaths

12th out-breath

On the 12th breath, the in-breath of inner space merges with the out-breath of outer space

Directionality and Bilaterality

The Maps of Outer and Inner Space of the Infinite

A through CCC deal with bilaterality or the map of the inner world

(Extract from Windows into Eternity)

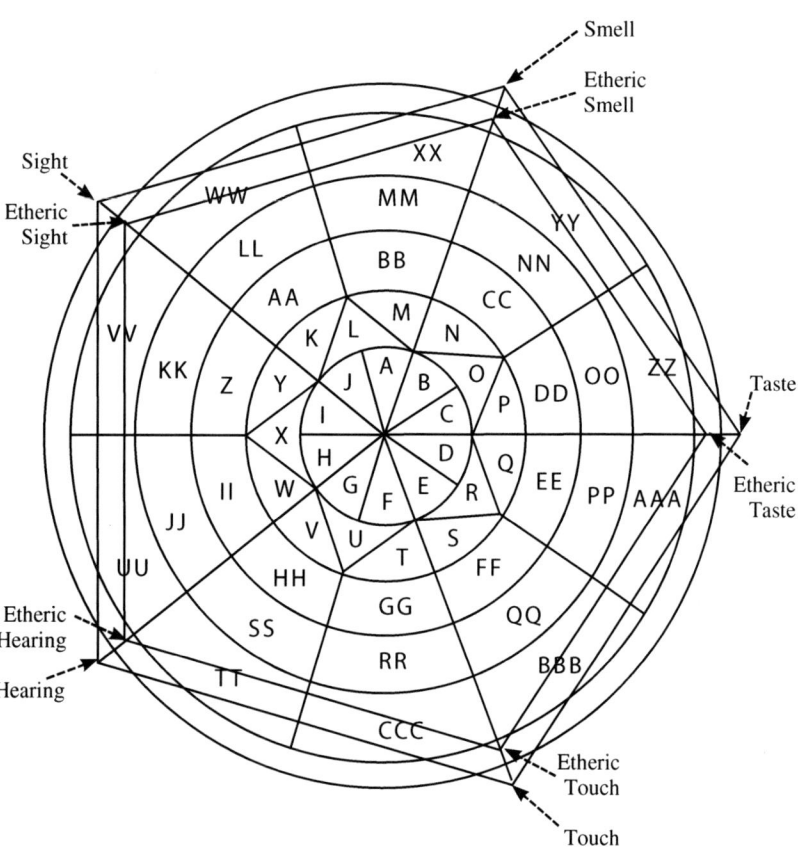

The five senses help determine direction, which is in turn determined by our map of outer space. The outer pentagon is the map for the five senses. The inner pentagon is the map for the 6th sense. Both deal with directionality, or directions and relationships of the outer world.

Key to the Maps of Space

The Emotional Pairs' Equations

A	Fulfillment	B	At-homeness
C	Innovation	D	Understanding
E	Flow	F	Appreciation
G	Learning	H	Exuberance
I	Triumph	J	Balanced Growth
K	Entertaining Journey	L	Accomplishment

The Pairs of States of Beings' Equations

M	Adoration	N	Joyous Journey
O	Enlightenment	P	Clarity of Vision
Q	Illumination	R	Divine Union
S	Inner Guidance	T	Divine Communion
U	Graceful Learning	V	Childlike Innocence
W	Regeneration	X	Discerned Living

The Pairs of Heart Energies' Equations

Y	Divine Compassion	Z	Reverence
AA	Pure Creativity	BB	Absolute Truth
CC	Impeccability	DD	Celebration
EE	Timing	FF	Focus
GG	Strength	HH	Grace
II	Clarity	JJ	Harmlessness

The Pairs of Physical Expressions' Equations

KK	Birth	LL	New birth
MM	Infinite Potential	NN	Sexual Communication
OO	Elation	PP	Discovery
QQ	Individuated Expression	RR	Faith
SS	Wonderment	TT	Joyous Accomplishment
UU	Divine Perfection	VV	Multi-faceted Acknowledgement

WW Through CCC are arrived at as follows:

WW = The total equation for + The total equation for
the Emotional Pairs   the States of Being

Heart Dance + Divine Heartsong = Ecstatic Embrace

WW = Ecstatic Embrace

XX = The total equation for + The total equation for
The States of Being   the Heart Energies

Divine Heartsong + Compassionate Understanding = Consecrated Living

XX = Consecrated Living

YY = The total equation for + The total equation for
the Heart Energies   the Physical Expressions

Compassionate Understanding + Rapture = Divine Love

YY = Divine Love

ZZ = The total equation for + The total equation for
the Emotional Pairs   the Heart Energies

Heart Dance + Compassionate Understanding = Self-sufficient Divinity

ZZ = Self-sufficient Divinity

AAA = The total equation for + The total equation for
the Emotional Pairs   the Physical Expressions

Heart Dance + Rapture = Cosmic Bliss

AAA = Cosmic Bliss

BBB = The total equation for + The total equation for
the States of Being   the Physical Expressions

Divine Heartsong + Rapture = Divine Rhapsody

BBB = Divine Rhapsody

CCC is the sum total of WW through to BBB. It is therefore the total of all frequencies on the map added together.

Ecstatic Embrace + Consecrated Living + Divine Love + Self-sufficient Divinity + Cosmic Bliss + Divine Rhapsody = Orgasmic Explosion of Love and Light

CCC = Orgasmic Explosion of Love and Light

The Keepers of the Seven Breaths

The Secret History of the Knowledge of Arasatma

The Gobekli Tepe People
Two Libraries, One Key

The Records of the Forgotten Ones

The Libraries of the Two Whales

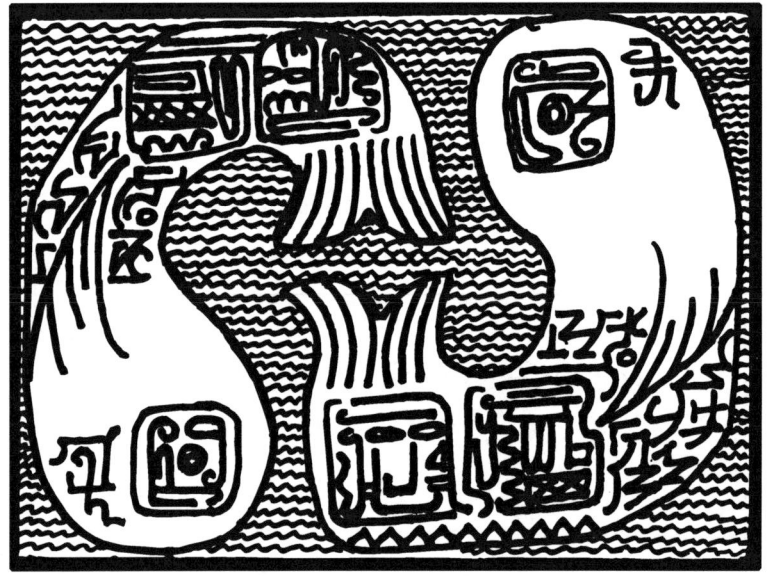

The Symbol For the Two Libraries

Secrets from the Libraries
of The Two Whales

Introduction

Chabech suve-uvatvi. Misevach utretva nanus kilsavat-hursta ubrakvi mina-uva-stachvavi.
Walk now the halls of records. To remember the story of the peoples of the Earth.

Bershpat urahak setva mishavach nestu. Isakve rustavi misech haresta nunavis herat ubasit mechnavi huras.
Remembrance is the first step to resolution. Only in remembering dreams can they be seen as the illusion that they are.

Nabach usu mishavat harshavat esekletve virastu blichvet birasachve hirustet. Nensevet ritva biruch aresta.
When the planet's history and secrets are suppressed, she becomes ill. Recalling dreams of long ago can help them be resolved and then forgotten.

Shivavet erseta mishavech ninsu elsatar pirasetvi harsvat mushech anasta. Kalsabi eresut haresta muvech blivaset.
The people of the buffalo stone will smoke their pipe to open the doors. Where the stone from heaven falls, is the place.

Kerech nesata arasatma esklavit.
Then shall the Arasatma Breaths be restored.

Glyphs from the Library of Two Whales

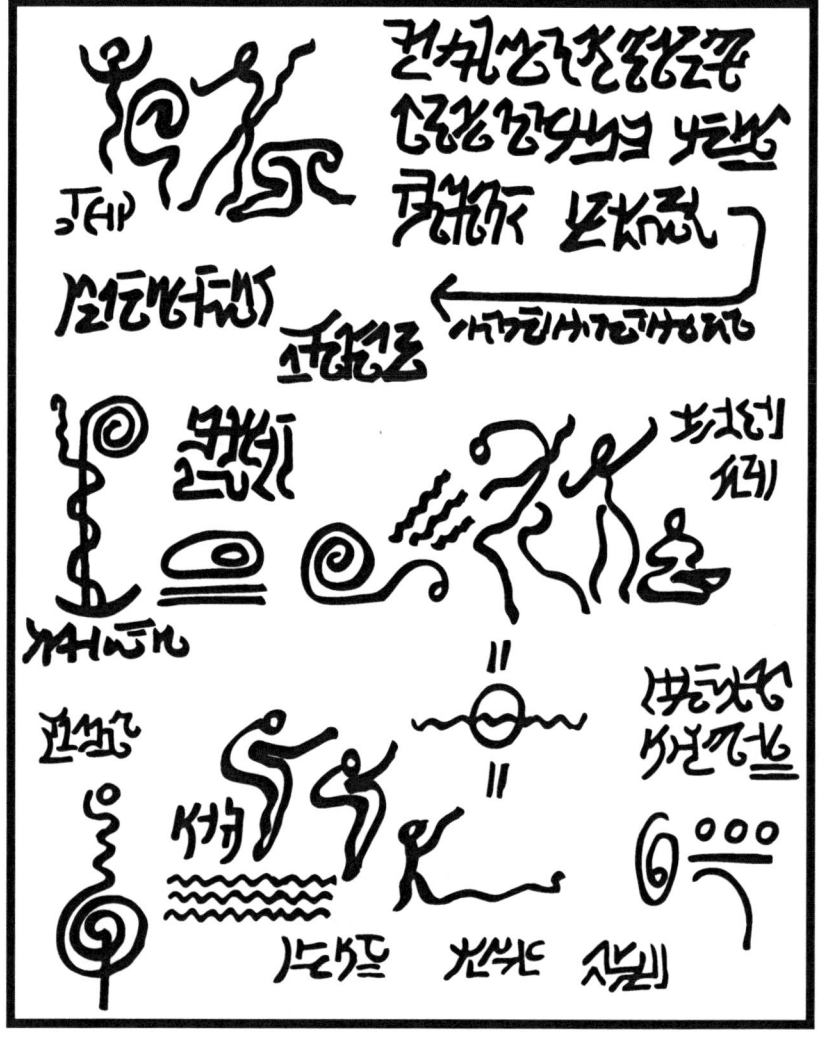

The Story of the Stone

Long ago when the Earth had lost its moon and a new moon was given in its place, designed to control the cycles of man, this story begins (75,000 years ago). The ancient tribes, seeing that a catastrophe would come, hid in the caverns of the crust of the Earth. Those who had lost the gift of prophecy did not and perished.

But a few, with powers long guarded from the eyes and ears of the profane, escaped another way. They were called the Whale Clan. They saw a tunnel in their dreams, that lead through the sky to a planet in the area of the Little Bear Star. They created long canoes, filled them with provisions and called upon the whales to guide them to the island where the tunnel was located.

Two whales came and led them to the island called Nanat Hestu Madal (Pohnpei Island in Micronesia), where they discovered ruins from the Ancient Ones – advanced beings who left before the previous catastrophe (about 200,000 years ago).

The Whale Clan saw the tunnel would lead them to Nanaktu, the Star of the Little Bear. They had to learn to sing with their bodies the same song as Nanaktu, and they would be pulled through the tunnel. Nanaktu would recognize their song and thinking them to be its children, call them home.

While they prepared themselves, they created records of what was, and what was to come. From the records comes a warning: When the Earth becomes too electrically charged, the magnetic fields decline. The poorly expressing magnetic (feminine) components and the over-emphasized electrical components (masculine) attract calamities. By grounding the electrical charges, life flourishes and calamities are either delayed or averted.

When the Whale Clan came to the island of Nanat Hestu Madal, they found in the ruins left behind by the Ancient Ones, writings on how to ground the electrical charges of the planet. They used this to delay the catastrophe long enough to prepare the records for those of the future to find, and so that they could change their frequency to match that on Nanaktu.

The Ancient Ones had created lagoons they stocked with electric eels and had built structures around them to ground the electricity. Where people around the Earth had knowledge of this, towers and obelisks were built to act as grounding rods. This caused the fields around them to flourish and the area to be less prone to weather disturbances.

Note: The round towers of Ireland have been noted to make the surrounding fields more productive. The early masons built them with a 3-degree taper, an extra degree of difficulty that provides significant benefit for antennas. These towers store magnetic and electromagnetic energy.

Among the records, the teachings of Arasatma, the Seven Breaths of Eternal Life, were found. The breaths would create within those who mastered them, indefinite longevity, power and the ability to avert catastrophes by using the pranic tube like a lightening rod.

When it was time for the Whale Clan to leave, seven men were chosen from among them to go back to the lands in the West carrying the records with them. They were given the gift of 'taytape' or timelessness so the long journey could be done in a short time.

They created the library to hold the records till it was the time for them to be found (on the Hobbema Indian Reserve, Alberta, Canada). Their powers were strong but their hearts were heavy as they bid farewell to their clan, for all could see that the tunnel would collapse when the times of trouble came.

When the records were safely hidden, they went into the Drum Mountain (Northern Montana, USA) to join the others of their people who hid there in the Earth. They were able to sustain themselves by catching the blind fish and eating water plants that were in the underground streams.

Some records were kept blank to be written upon when the Earth's time of pain was over. The prophecies had said that a wolf would come to tell when it was safe to leave. These records (along with others that had been brought from the islands) would also be hidden in the library until it was time for them to be released from their caverns.

The library of the two whales would lie undetected until the time would come when the stone would fall from the sky. One would come who will see it fall – the beginning of the opening of the knowledge of the libraries would then be near.

Note: The meteorite was seen falling from the sky by a man from the Hobbema reserve. He dug it up and showed it to Almine when she came to Red Deer. She heard it speak of the two libraries of the Two Whales and the Bear. It was only after a small group of native Cree people from the Hobbema reserve held a pipe ceremony on the spot where the meteor had fallen, that the libraries, located on the site beneath the ground, began yielding their secrets. The Cree are the original keepers of the secrets of the breaths.

Excerpts from the Original Records of the Ancient Ones

I. Charuk Anekvi Harasta

Persva Nektu elesvi manech

Reksa parus ustavi helasvi

Neksaru brivatet ereksa

Walasu nisat ikperenus vravi

Mechtu nensach hublavesvi

Ekbaru neksavi vibrechvi

Klasut isat michter harasut

Erekne sichvet subla vesvi

Nektaru hiraspahur nisarut

Espa blihet sparavek ublavi

Kisanat herstu minavech sabaru

Nechklarut hurut sabarechvi

Ikret velstan misut araksta

Herset velchspi biranesvi urat

Kanuch husanit pirekspavi

2. Irksabaru Huvetspi Ananach

Netret bilarus arsapa minavi

Kesba pires arsata miselanach huret

Ekbar suklabit viselvi anas

Sukpavit hursava vivavach anus

Priset kletvatra bishet

Kesenach blisparet misenet uras

Karut bilsprakta herenas usit

Arsanu itrek blavatvi misavech

Pletpranut harsta ukretvi

Mananut hursba eksaltu

Kavavis mispach blivabespi

Sparut eklahus hereshtek vivespi

Setrebit akla veravish nenachtu

Arasat brivet arkpava hikranus blivaspi

Retrachbavi hiravat sikret enenus

3. Mirshpava iretsatu Nineklat-pravi

Mechbi sursarat arekla bravi

Retvi huravespi miravek arktu

Isevech mishbaret hiruklet sarsavi

Nechbaruk urspe kerenus-vava

Visetrech pliset arektu vivas

Hustanavit irekpla britbravi

Kisunet arkpa miset herehusvi

Ketrebis-barut misel virk parva

Haraktu misech pavi aras

Asanet kavavi-vanush hirasvi

Isel privatur hisanach usetvarvi

Prubavat arkvi neneklut

Kusel nistru briharsanot urakvi

Abarut sihet itrevi minuvech

Arkarut nekvi blishet arstu

4. Ush nenska hurit valshparva

Karik nenesklu pars pranit uben

Suktaher vilespavi aretrabahur sursa

Nikpar nenskla hirsavet utrech

Resatu nerechvi aras tretvavi

Sitkluher bilasat renek harasklu

Iskanut eklever resenetvi

Siklu erksavir sechvavi

Huret manivar itrek barusnevi

Spibach eseklu sahit aresta

Kubit sitremanur urasani

Kinisat helestruch bitrenut

Arat plibahur nektavis sutranit

Spibar siklet pravi varavis

Stuchna spelehurs-plavik

Litranasur munet balavi sekva

The Grounding of Electrical Energy by Individuals

Light was created when the first analyses of experience took place. Frequency was created to retain in memory that which needed to be understood. This created the first illusion: That anything can be known. When everything can be called a 'new expression' in every moment, the way the ocean is never the same twice but yet an eternal existence, anything 'known' is but the holding onto of an obsolete truth.

Light is but accessed knowledge – electricity in action. The addiction to light comes from the fear and pain that arises as we imagine ourselves to be trapped in our self-made maze of questions and answers. We seek within the maze for the answer on how to get out of it. We assuage the feeling of being lost by always seeking the next answer, which always begets the next question.

In aware experience without interpretation, all desire to interpret is left behind. The electric, mind-based individual, having changed his need to seek understanding to effortless knowing, becomes like a grounding rod. Life flourishes in the presence of such a being and catastrophic change becomes unnecessary.

Cherez araska-hit arkla berenut plech parhu ninas erskleresve.
Release now the trauma held in the over-burdened memories of the feminine.

Mechtu-sihat uvespe spiharut nich ve mines parspara ararat varis.
Through the expression of the poetry in your heart are past wounds healed.

Bispa erech uhuru-rasvahit mista uranes.
Only then will all questions cease.

The Library of the Two Whales

The knot of the thread of time is held in the libraries of the Two Whales. As it opens, the thread of time will begin to unravel (2012).

Note: The Mayan calendar has predicted that time in its linear form will end in 2012.

Time is the movement of awareness in the space opened between a question and an answer. The Library of the Bear is also upon the place of the People of the Buffalo Stone. It lies within the ancient hills of the Bear Claw and holds the knot of space. When time changes, so does space. Live now the life of no questions and the Bear Libraries will open their secrets to you.

Writing from the Library of Two Whales I

Writing from the Library of Two Whales 2

The People of the Bear Clan

Insights from the Scrolls of Hansarat

Insights into the Eternal Dance
From the Scrolls of Hanasat

Chirach mesete hunasvi sklarak
Prihesta vibrech suherestat unach

Believe in nothing, for only then can you freely and effortlessly know.

Spiharach nesetu biresh privahet bires esekle huset. Virsabach uretvi
karus pares minevesvi sekre utret paravi.

Seek not meaning, for it retains that which has become meaningless.
Perception without conclusion brings clarity.

Brinavik usechvi mishet henasech brihet vibrech sparetvi nensarat husple ustavi vibrachvi minuvit.

As long as the judgment of good and bad exists, dictators will arise to defend or enforce their point of view.

Mechpa nanuset herevesh arastu blivech sarsatu uhuvaset nusta habaset hurespi.

Inspiration does not come in the form of an idea, but as a subtle, yet profound change in the song of your life.

Shivahet ubrechvi minusat ekles harasparvi minech savatu shelehes vavit ekratbi minahes.

Do not fear pain, for it is in pushing through and beyond it that you will find greater joy.

Michta brisabek erekte-vi aras menetu plivechvi hersata minaves brivabek herestu anach selsava priviravech anesviva.

Individuations are the seekers of self-beauty and wonderment within the eternal, undifferentiated flow of existence.

Kersavach minusuch brivat herespi aklatva herestu minasuch vibresvi arasut. Nechspahur esekletvi mishtahur enestravi erech pahur nanunes.

In speaking mind-to-mind, or even heart-to-heart, we speak the shallow words of deception. No two perspectives can converse, as the perspective of each is unique.

Nansklave misevech hunavesvi eruret blihavech eskre bravet sklava prihanes eresh asatu minevat skaravink.

Let your words flow from the eternal silence of your infinite song, that the depth of your being may touch that of another between your words.

Mesetu misanech herstu mishal arek navesbi plivahet eklestru mavech vilestra pravekvi eres nanustra. Kiva hes esetra mivavechspri arunas uvahespi.

No separation can exist, therefore no relationship. The Infinite does not express or there would be a relationship between the expressed and the expresser. There is no such thing as creation; there is only the One Life.

Shebevich neskave prihat minasut blives estreve unas herspata vibrachvi sklerut aresta. Plihes nenes harspava vibrech sta-unit ereklesve virsh prahut nenechvi stahuvit aresta spivarech neneshtavu pli-es.

Speak not to manipulate, control or persuade, but let your words be free from attached outcome. Your words are the veils that are drawn to reveal or conceal the never-ending mysteries of the Eternal Being.

Kirsava herestu minuvech vibrasvi ersaklut uras pirit uklet vibrasvi harsata ustech nunes blivabas arska. Krives nichvetur harsata mishenuch ubret prahasvi verenuch sahabit arevestu aranach.

Taste becomes an addiction when it is used as a substitute to fill the gaps left by deprivation of touch. Explore your world with touch to receive its sacred alchemy of inspiration.

Kelspahur sklehura nespava virsprechvu nanunish esekle prehut. Virsenech herus arsatva misech haruhet privavet vibech kranas suvit erekletvi minach hersetu vibret arunas klaharuvit vibret eres usta blivechvi verespa ste-unit.

Touch is the way to explore life in a deeper way. Allow yourself to feel with more than your skin, for in feeling an object, or another with the fullness of your being, alchemy of inspired, exponential change occurs.

*Kelshavich visetret unas bliverevichva uhur nispavek vibrech sta-
uharanit stelenechvi varsatur esenit kenuch virevespahur eselvi
archpahur minavish hersetu skravele vispahur nuvataa uresvi.*

Be aware of what food you wish to reach for, since it serves the
purpose through taste, of inspiring into expression the full resonance
of the indivisible and eternal that you are.

Neksavu vibrechvi anas eres ukletvi berech baruk mishe netvi hersatu.

There is no meaning to primal existence, just the Eternal Self
observing Itself.

Sikrat nurnavi erekta plavabit arsanach set vileshva hurspahur
nechta skrevileveshvi misenech setur na skri-uhurunat valeshvi
uherevi. Nantach bires etrevanik beletre nanuchvra bilestur subatu
mishenechvi.

Eating is a sacred ritual that fulfills its holy purpose only in the silence
of thoughtful contemplation, gratitude and sensitive awareness. The
sense of taste inspires the notes of the Eternal Song.

Kriharavit peleshestravi minach sivatur meshpavi ersetur hiravachvi
blisbabek ekre suhat perevesvi unet. Santuvi-es kriharavishvi
nanutach prihestravu skrihavet nanustar.

The appreciative eyes of the master reveal the hallowed sacredness
of life. The eyes of one who thinks he knows, affirm the shallow
illusions of life.

Selevish akratprahur sechva nestu haravis praheretat skriha-uvi nenech suhar privesvi. Karchsavu minevit plihesvi araksta brivabech heres ursata viselenut selevishna-es.

Sight is a doorway through which the real and eternal enters to perceive Itself. When sight believes it knows, it creates its own prison bars of belief systems.

Ursetpravahur nenek hiresta bravich eres kletvravir belestachvi nersba huretur pleva.

When the real touches the real, rapture results and all of reality changes.

Nersklerut erektrachvi virseblat minusech heres urstava blishet prehat areklatvi stra-uhes birseta. Rachnet bri-eklatur siberutpavi misenut havravesbi skelanot. Esklerut prehana sebevich estet manuvit.

The four matrices of existence through which life rotates, and which in man form the body, soul and spirit, were themselves formed when sight, hearing, feeling and touch separated from functioning as a whole. Smell never fell into separateness.

The People of the Bear Clan

When the travail of the Earth was past and the wolf called the people of the Buffalo Stone home, the libraries of the Two Whales and the Library of the Bear were opened in a gathering of the elders. In a most sacred meeting, the ancient songs were sung after a fast of four days and four nights had been observed by the people. The elders in a holy lodge received visions and spoke to their departed ancestors about the records they had received from the Ancient Ones they called Mana-tu.

A spirit of great radiance, a woman, appeared and taught them the seven holy breaths of Arasatma. She said that the power of the breaths were only for the pure in heart who had surrendered his or her own needs to the Creator. The ability to walk in multiple realities at once would come to those who mastered the breaths and therefore the records had to be protected.

She taught the elders how to use the full pranic tube that reaches into the Earth and that they would become as a pipe that would ground heaven and Earth. The records had to be divided into seven breaths and taken by seven men into their own libraries and into distant lands.

The 5th breath, The Breath of the Fire Walk, would be kept in the Bear Library and the 6th breath, The Breath of the Divine Marriage, would be kept in the Libraries of the Two Whales. She would guide the five who travelled to distant lands in their dreams if they walked in reverence upon the Earth.

The people would be taught the sacred pipe ceremony to communicate with the Creator. Only the few would know that it was a reminder that through the extended use of the pranic tube, the holy pipe can become ourselves.

The young men who went their way were never heard of again but their story of how they carried the breaths of the 'pipe' to the distant lands was told for many generations around the fires of the people as they spread across the lands.

An Example of the Glyphs from the Libraries of the Two Whales

The Story of the Ancient Ones

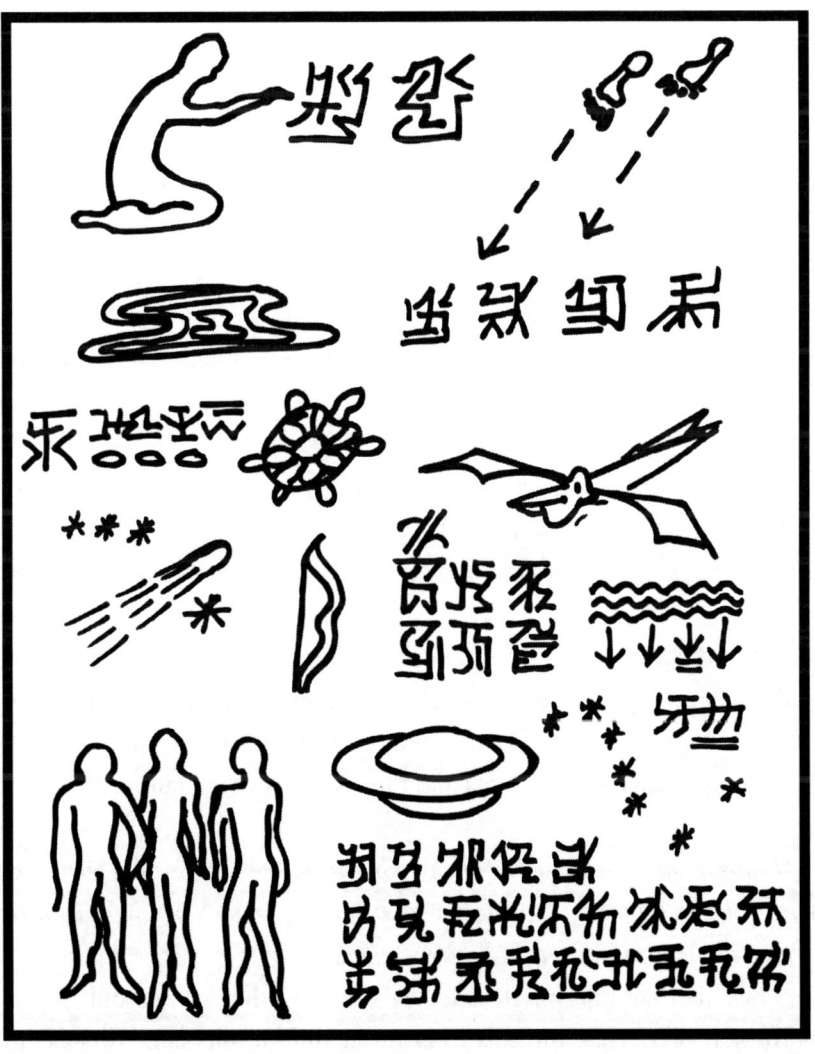

The Yaravet – Singers of the Wolf Song

Kee pah anas seve utranis pah husne utre kiharanat vi uklet. Sinaya sipahu nesva atrunat sehit akla nanunis harstruva aya.

From the northlands (Northeastern Russia) came a strange people of the wolf clan. Their clothes were spun like a spider's web of many bright colored threads.

Chahuba asana kiras estavi minach harsatu kiras piraha nusta ekle virabas esna uhustu peraret. Kiya michta blivaset erastu kiva sihestra misenachve setve resta mispa aklanit hirasat vibrachtu minavis.

They made the journey across the bridge of ice to seek new lands after the destruction came to their lands. Tame wolves lived with them and they made music on a string like we used for our bow to shoot arrows.

Nansaru kihi-eeya savatu menech sehus asatva kivarus arsta birut aret nunach sa hatva uhinya. Kerese bi-atra misha nunavas hersetu arsta keresutva ahanutva ruvitva rekvatu manis areyastava rutva hivastu.

They made markings on bark and skins to communicate (writing) and left drawings in caves where they gathered for stories. They made permanent marks (tattoos) on their bodies to tell the stories of the important events of their lives and their status in the clan.

Paarch nuset arasta harunekva blivaset harastu esenet erta ukla virsavet priyanunesvi. Arstahur sich havet plesut harstava visenasvi arakstar birahus parvet arch bavis vavet.

They had strange magic and walked upon hot stones but did not burn their feet. They did this to bring healing to the sick and ease the pain of birth while the women sang in trembling, high tones.

Karsu achna biset harstava brivet arak sarsatu. Krivasat misbech erste harus krivaves harsatu michba.

When they danced they did so in male and female pairs. The women put flowers in their long braided hair.

Taruk arsata michbanaru hereta. Skirarut viset blivabech menehuspavi ares tuhayehetvavi mishbahur. Reksatu misevech viraset haranus ekresutravit harasta.

Their hair was black but their skin pale. The women were prized for the roundness of their face and form. The men hunted with spears, bows and knives for food.

Esta Yaravet misuheresat arsta nunuk helebrut uras esteve miras nuchbere harat nanusta.

Thus the Yaravet came to live on our lands and at night their wolves sang to the wild ones.

The Yaravet and the Sacred Breath

When the Yaravet came to our lands, seven generations had passed since the people came out of the crust of the Earth. They lived in peace among our people at a distance that allowed us to go our separate ways. It was not until the eighth generation was born that a man named Taruk came from the Yaravet and asked, with gestures of his hands, to stay among us and study our ways and language.

When he had learned to speak our tongue, he was able to explain that he was a holy man called Pa-a-ro, which means in his tongue: Keeper of the Breath. He said that many generations ago, one that looked like the People of the Buffalo Stone, had come across the land bridge to teach them the 3rd breath, The Breath of Heaven and Earth, the breath of the belly.

He showed us a rolled-up skin that showed a man of our people holding a tablet. He wanted to know the story of the breaths and teach our elders the breath kept by the Yaravet. A few of the elders among us yet had the knowledge of all seven breaths. For years Taruk stayed among us and carried the knowledge of the 5th and 6th breath, as well as the 3rd breath, held by the Yaravet. Eventually, he returned to his people to share his knowledge.

The Imaru – People of the Long Boats

Keepers of the Breath of the Fountain of Life - the Seventh Breath

From the oral traditions of the Toltec mystics, there was a native tribe in Florida massacred between 300 and 350 years ago. Much of their wisdom, gained from the study of the Breath of the Fountain of Life, perished with them. They had lived in what is now Mexico until about 2,000 years ago, when 'a strange star in the sky' caused massive upheavals. They then moved into the Florida area.

They resisted writing because they felt it solidified the flow of the breath around the body and caused static belief systems that imprisoned us. The oral traditions tell that they created very long boats from reeds and were experts at water travel.

The Imaru had fled from a 'feathered shadow god' who taught the people of the Azteka how to do black magic in his name, using blood sacrifice. He also taught them how to steal the souls of the dead. This caused conquerors to come to the lands.

The Imaru escaped the black magicians by leaving their native lands. They had preyed upon the Imaru because they knew that somehow they held powerful abilities and knowledge. The Imaru died keeping the secret of the Breath of the Fountain of Life safe.

The Avi-atara – People of the Bird Tribes

Keepers of the Breath of the Winged Ones – the Second Breath

From the Records of the Libraries of the Falcon, located in Mongolia.

We write in stone our story that one day the tale of our people will be read when they are as dust upon the Earth and their memory is whispered only on the wind. We go gladly to our ancestors for we are as the snow that melts to feed the great river of life. But we pass to those with eyes to see, our most sacred possession: the Sacred Breath of the Winged Ones.

In our stone tablets lie its secrets, entrusted to us by the emissary of the Holy Mother. They shall be sealed in the secret cave and guarded by the spirit of the Great Falcon until the time that one shall come that can call them forth and read their words. When these records are again opened, it shall be known as *The Time of the Gathering*. In those days shall the Ancient Ones again walk on the Earth as though they are men. Then shall the knowledge of the Sacred Breaths be gathered from their fallen keepers of the four directions. But a few of these once powerful nations shall remain and fewer still shall find these truths.

The Avi-atara lived in the fertile valley of the Great Serpent River (where India joins Asia and the Himalayas now stand). We were in harmony with the land and our spirits were strong. We knew that the Earth would be struck by the great mountain from the sky and in their dreams the wise ones among us, known as the Avitars, saw that the race must be preserved.

Far to the North, a natural tunnel into the crust of the Earth was seen in the visions of the wise ones. As many couples as there are fingers and toes travelled there on the fastest horses to escape the coming cataclysm. The devastation was worse than what could have been imagined. Where millions had lived in a fertile river valley, the lands had collided and mountains arose. The few Avi-atara that returned home now had to live on top of the roof of the world.

It was a magic man with feathers hanging from his hair that brought us the Breath of the Winged Ones. Not long after he taught it to us, he lay down and died. We knew his heart was heavy with longing for his people and he wished to walk with the ancestors as a spirit: to be reborn among his kin.

We created a library to keep the holy truths and the story of the Avi-atara, the People of the Bird Tribes. Never again shall our culture die without leaving a footprint in time. Thus we entrust those of you who will know our words' truth, to tell our story around the fires in days to come.

The People of Ashwantu
The Ancient Lands (Ethiopia)

Keepers of the Breath of the Lion's Gate – the First Breath

In the catastrophes of the Earth, there are a few places that seemed to be able to remain undisturbed. The Earth herself, known to us as Alamana (the word means 'of everyone, or all, the Mother's), must have decreed that it be so. Our land has stood firm when others sank. Even when the Earth herself trembled in agony, did our land stand firm. We were here when the invaders came from Habiru (known in the Sumerian records as the planet Nibiru), and when they left, we were still upon these lands. (The word Hebrew came from Habiru. The Star of Bethlehem was actually Nibiru – which comes close to Earth every 3,000 years.)

Lineages of those initiated as High Priests have been the custodians of the many secrets we have kept. But none more prized than the secret of the Breath of the Lion's Gate. The mastery of this breath was prized and studied for many years. There were multiple levels of proficiency and when reached, enabled the master to wear upon his person the sacred symbol designating his particular level of mastery.

The Lion's gate (the pineal gland, the pituitary and the hypothalmus) can be used as a stargate when the breath is fully mastered; something that becomes more possible during specific phases of the conjunction of Sirius with the Earth and the moon. This allows the ability to communicate with beings from other planets and to study their planetary civilizations.

The history of how the breath came to our lands is lost in antiquity. We know only that it happened when the lands of Khem (Egypt) were still flooded and that it was brought by an old man who had travelled very far from the East.

When the invaders' children and grandchildren were born upon the Earth, their lifespans were much shorter. With each generation it became more so. They trampled our land looking for the sacred mushroom that looks like a phallus. It has the ability to prolong life for about 1,000 years.

The mushroom and the water vegetable that youthens were given to us by the Holy Mother and where they grow is a secret we keep.

It is not from the past we speak, as we bring our knowledge for the long awaited gathering of the breaths. We practice and guard the Breath of the Lion's Gate still and speak mind to mind.

It was many generations later, after we had received the Breath, that a bald man in yellow robes came to us from the East. He brought to us the Breath of the Little Horn. He asked only that we teach him the Breath we guarded. His name was Nafti.

Nafti had seen that another cataclysm would come in the future (9,564 BC) and that our lands would not perish. The land of his origin was called the Land of Gems. It was occupied by a shadow 'goddess' who used the science of Habiru and black magic to subdue the people. He was the last to carry the knowledge of the breath – the others had been killed.

He had seen our lands in a vision and was surprised that they were in the shape of the little horn at the base of the spine. The Breath of the Little Horn and the Breath of the Lion's Gate could be used together to decrease density and slow down time. His heart knew we would keep the 4th breath as safe as we kept the 1st.

Note: The mushroom mentioned were very rare and only known by a few people. They were originally found in Ethiopia, but are no longer available. Also due to the heavy radiation in our air and water from nuclear reactor meltdowns and resulting radiation leakage, sea vegetables have become contaminated. The best alternative is Klameth lake blue-green algae.

The Symbols of Mastery
From Ethiopia

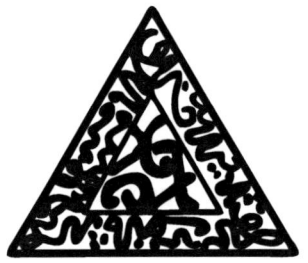

1. The enjoyment of life's unfoldment

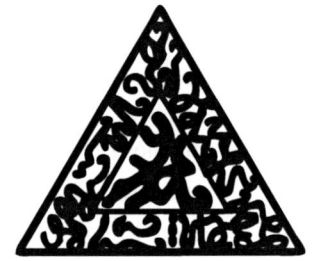

2. The freedom of authentic living

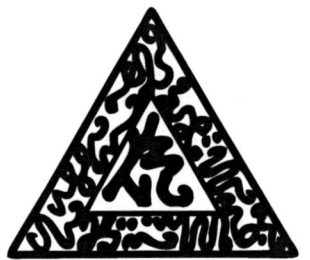

3. The power of alignment

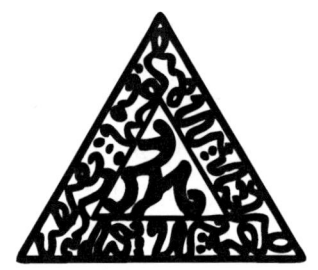

4. The surrender to the One life

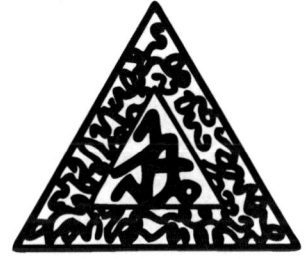

5. Trusting the perfection

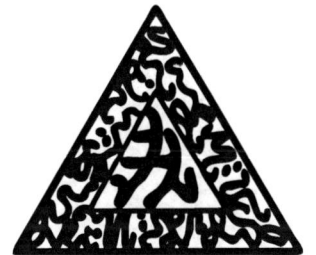

6. Abundant resources

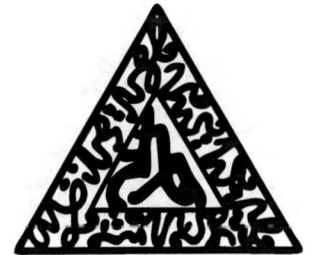

7. Restoration of youth

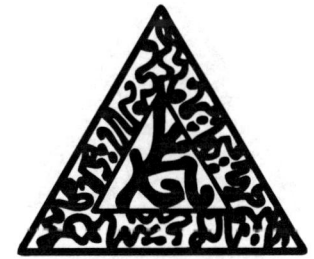

8. Enhancing beauty

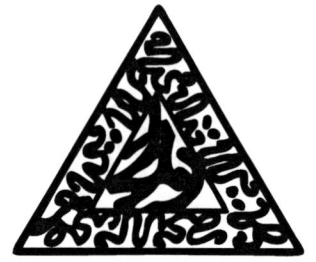

9. Freedom from illusion

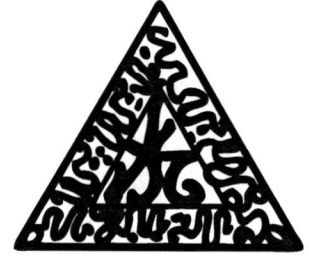

10. Grace and elegance

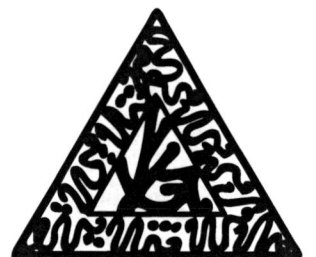

11. Rapture and bliss

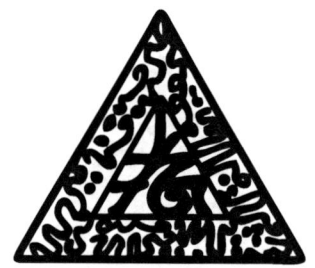

12. Increase through
gratitude

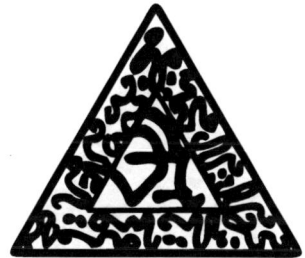

13. Love in expression

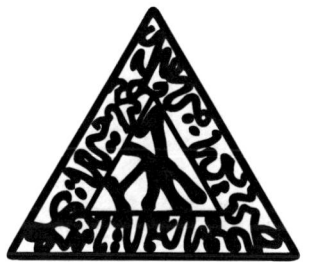

14. Praise and jubilation

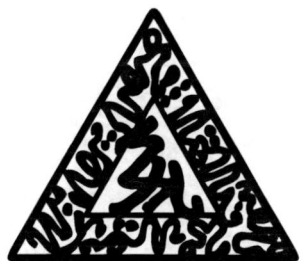

15. Peace and tranquility

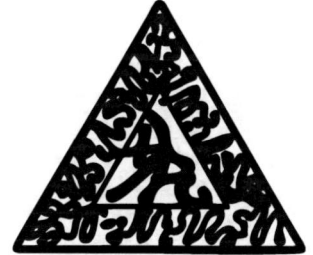

16. The manifestation of
     absolute truth

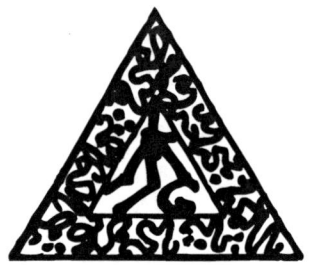

17. Recognition of the divine

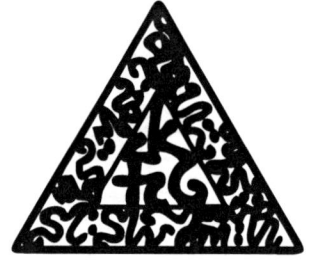

18. Releasing all paradigms

19. Joyous adventure

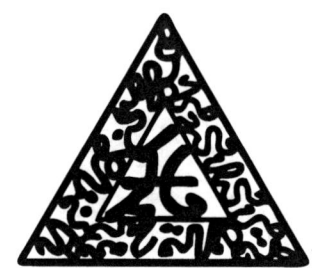

20. Transcending mortal boundaries

Closing

The greatest light has always shone on Earth at the time of greatest darkness. And so it is that wondrous tools of great power and life-changing gifts are available at this time when the burdens of humanity seem to have increased as well.

No longer hidden in mystery, no longer only available to the few who tread the hallowed halls of temples; they come to us openly, available to all who are able to recognize their inestimable worth. They speak to those who resonate to their holiness, even when they are not wrapped in the trimmings associated with the sacred.

May the openness of our hearts allow them to release their gifts to us. To the glory of the One Life and Its wondrous expressions as the many, forever and ever.

BOOK TWO

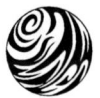

Nevi-Satma
The Twelve Breaths of Proxy

Breathing Techniques to
Cleanse Radiation from the Body

*Through the use of the ancient symbols
of Barachstan, the body's cleansing can
become a proxy for removing radiation from
the waters of the Earth...*

Introduction to the Nevi-Satma, the Twelve Breaths of Proxy

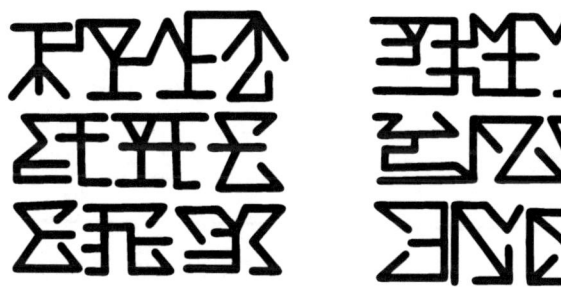

From the long-forgotten northeastern lands of Lemuria, called Barachstan, come symbols of power. These ancient symbols once used for water magic, create a link between the one and the many, allowing the purification of the body to become a powerful proxy for the waters of the Earth.

At a time when radiation is affecting the water table of the Earth, we have been given the breathing techniques as a means of purifying the Earth and her resources. The 34 concepts are to be studied before practicing the 12 Breaths of Proxy. They provide the necessary perception to help effect a profound but subtle change in the clarity and purity of our emotions – a prerequisite for cleansing the fluids of the body.

Note: It is an important prerequisite that prior to doing the Nevi-Satma, Twelve Breaths of Proxy, you have practiced and completed all 3 Levels of the Arasatma Breaths. Level III should be completed at least 3 times before doing the Nevi-Satma Breaths.

See Appendix IV for information on *Creating Sacred Space* and *Working with Sacred Wheels*.

The 34 Concepts to Purify the Emotions for the Twelve Breaths of Proxy

The Wheel of Purification

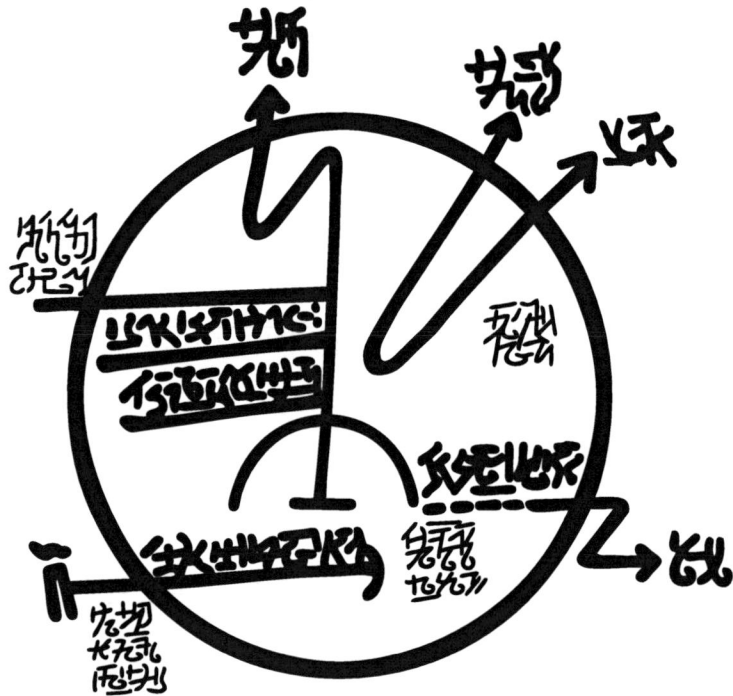

Cleansing radiation from the bloodstream, will cleanse
the radiation from the waters of the Earth.

1. An pe kihang nin xavi

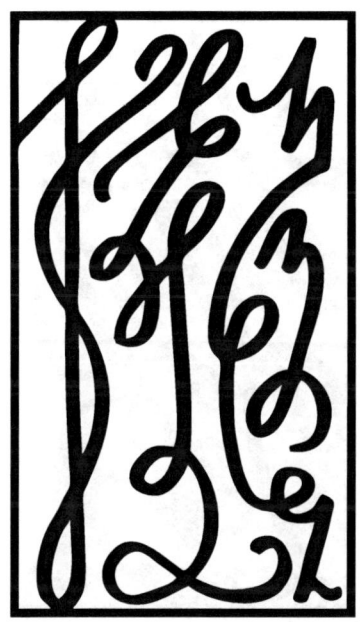

Only that which the moment contains can fill the cup of our happiness. All else is but a nostalgic dream colored by the longing to return to the obsolete high points of yesterday.

2. Burutat yanang setevi

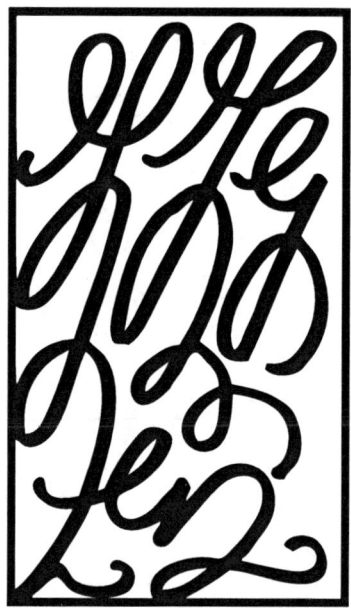

The one who is not at home within the contentment of his being, will search for eternity to find the elusive element to bring the fulfillment that eludes him. In grateful acknowledgement for the blessings the moment brings, lies the bounty of a fulfilled life.

3. Sinasat xianang sparut

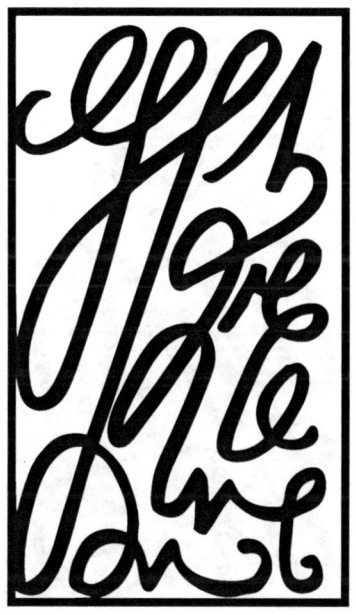

In our creative contribution to the quality of the moment, do we chisel from the unhewn rock of time, a fulfilled life of poise and grace? In asking what we can get from the moment, we deplete both our environment and ourselves.

4. Kina sutat blihanan

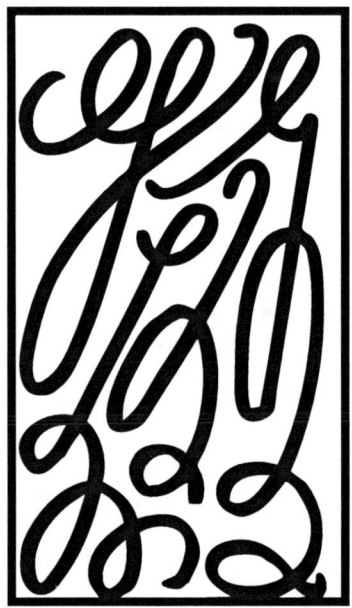

In yearning for 'what next' instead of appreciating 'what is', we rob the fulfillment of our future dreams of the foundation upon which to build them. The future is shaped by the moment well-lived. The abandonment of the moment leads to the haphazard and graceless formation of the future.

5. *Biristat kelsanan kiranit senotang*

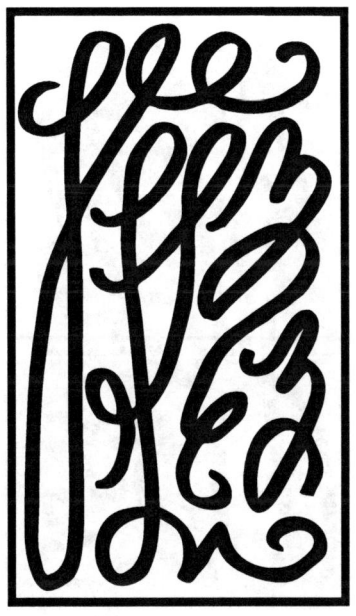

Grateful acknowledgement of the gifts the moment brings, ensures their presence in even greater abundance in the future. This is based on the ability of each being to contribute to the quality of the moment by what is emphasized through our attitudes, emotions and focus.

6. *Kipanun evevi kihanang asata*

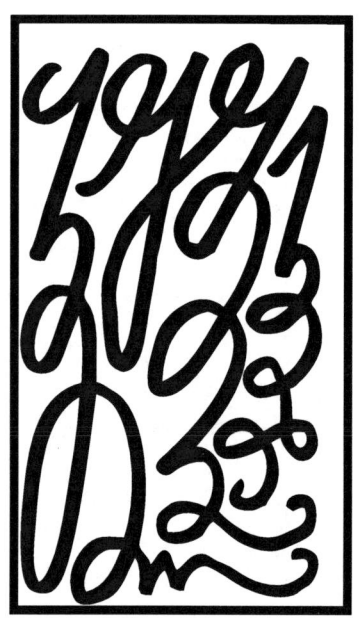

Linear time is a bewildering concept to an eternal being. The core of each being is timeless, even though it is obscured by the layers of personality that have accumulated like dust through the ages. In not understanding the nature of this illusion, we become its victim. We believe ourselves to be transient, like a moment of expression within eternal time, when we do not understand that there is only one eternal moment stretching throughout eternity.

7. *Vinayeng suti mishang nanut*

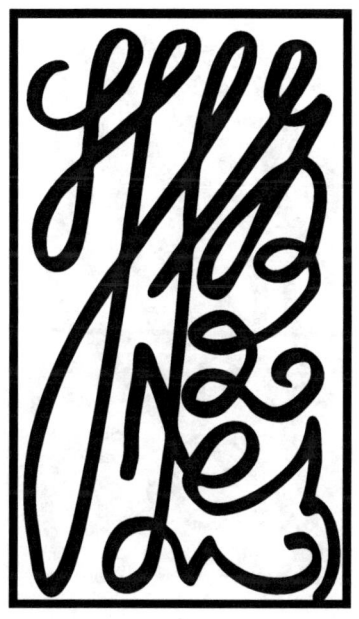

We spend a great deal of resources trying to help others achieve the same level of happiness we have. But happiness comes from awareness of present blessings. If the awareness is not there, increasing the blessings for another will not be able to bring happiness beyond just a fleeting moment of gladness.

8. Blisat pavet erseneng hurihat satayang

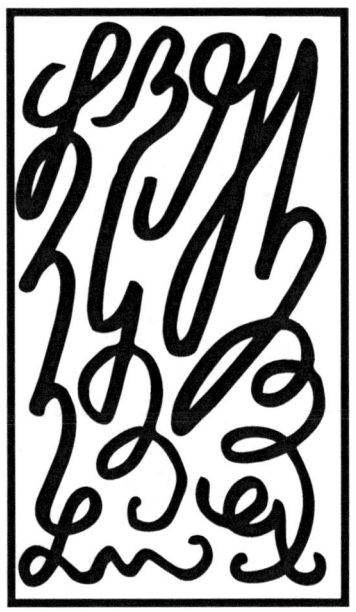

Achievement without a sense of accomplishment is hollow. Chasing achievement without allowing yourself to enjoy its gifts, is like running after the wind. Acknowledge your accomplishments, for within them you can observe the illuminated aspects of your being in action.

9. Kihura satet pishaneng utu

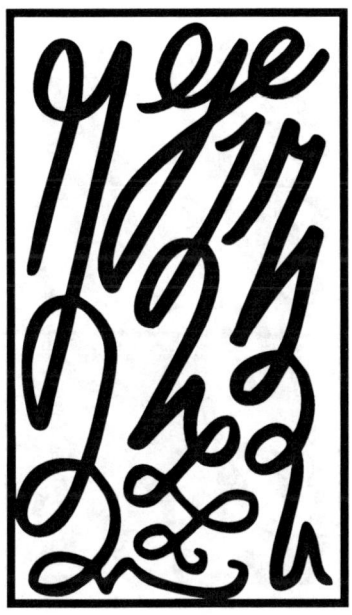

Being bound by yesterday's standards, through the nostalgic value given to them by the heart, prevents even greater achievements today. When we value the high points of the past as a springboard for even greater things to come, they fulfill their purpose as the inspiration for the excellence of the moment.

10. Kelvi ara satsanun hersetay

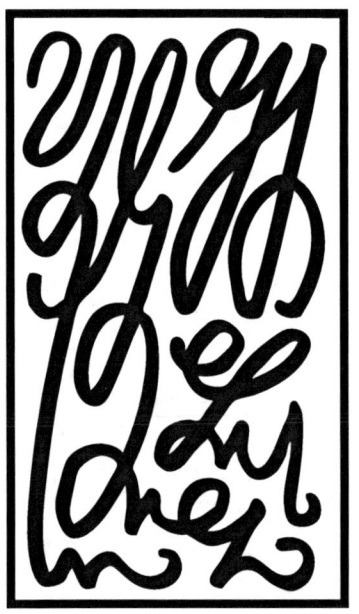

One of the greatest enslavements of man is the imposing of external value systems on him. Any value system of what is praiseworthy and what is not, only considers superficial appearances. The vast riches of the inner life are not accounted for, nor the fact that under the law of compensation, the inner withers when the external is overemphasized. Take time for deep, meaningful living that the actions of your life may be weighed by the deep satisfaction and joy that they bring.

11. Akva nesheng xi-ang vava

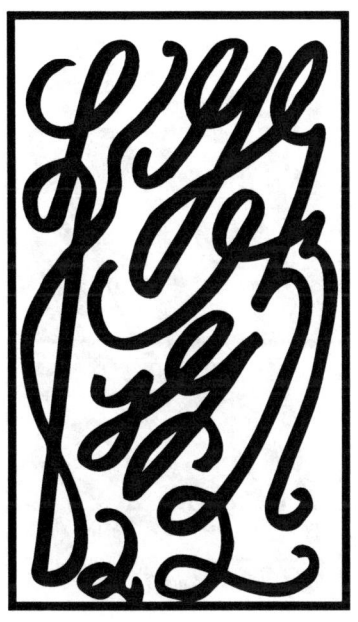

Gratitude is a primary impetus for increasing abundance. Yet gratitude cannot exist in the presence of expectation and a sense of entitlement. Do not base gratitude for your blessings on comparisons. In seeing that you have more because another has less, you make of him your opposite. The law of opposites decrees that because the increase of one is determined by the decrease of another, there is a debt that has been incurred and must be repaid.

12. Plishenen subita ananeng

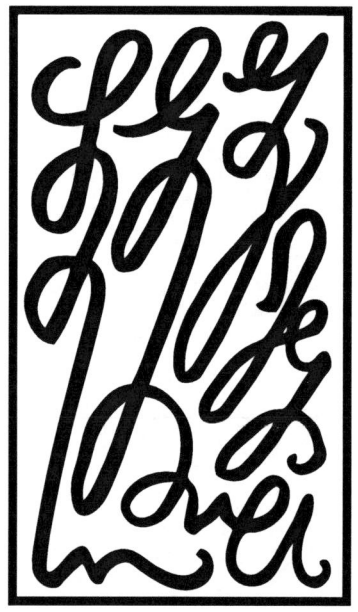

The egoic self is an arbitrary reference point within the vastness of our eternal being, from which we choose to experience the discovery of ourselves. Our familiarity with a specific reference point has created the false impression that we are that specific point of view, rather than the limitlessness of our true being. But each day can be lived from whatever reference point we choose in order to experience ourselves. We change the reference point by changing our attitudes and focus.

13. Viras peres savi miteni

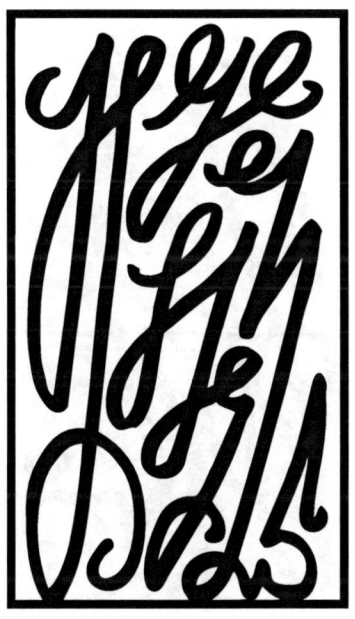

When the pressure of a crisis situation is encountered, the tendency is to regress to the coping mechanisms of the past. This causes an obsolete reaction to the situation, rather than a masterful response. An overwhelming situation can only be surmounted by surrendering to the eternal knowing of our being and allowing our actions to flow automatically.

14. *Karasung sinan elklevi arus*

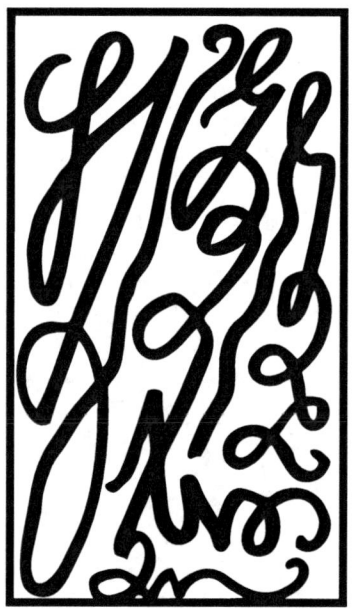

Leadership as a quality is highly valued among men. But it is frequently the result of the greatest arrogance of all: the belief that we can know anything for sure. Those who deduce the present based on the past do not consider that behind the face value of life, all is continually renewed. The only one who has anything of worth to impart, is he or she who, by embracing the unfathomability of life, allows the miracle of new unfoldings to express effortlessly through themselves.

15. Kespanun esekle brivabus

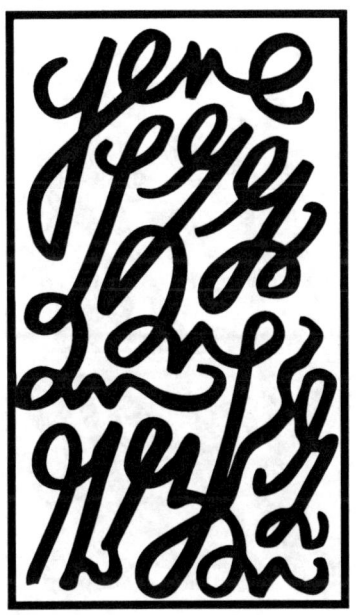

Many fear what they deem to be undesirable traits within themselves. The usual coping mechanism is to suppress them. But suppression breeds virility, and thus the suppressed traits will eventually break free with far more strength than they had before. This creates even more suppression. The fear of these traits will disappear when we learn that we can masterfully choose what impulses we express, observing the rest without judgment, allowing them to rise and fall like the waves of the deep ocean.

16. Aknang selhet usetvi anasu

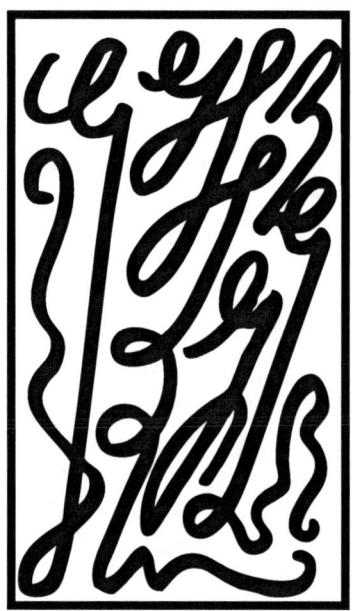

The rejection of others can be the impetus of excellence or the fuel for the self-destructive fire of victimhood. Excellence, by definition, is that which rises beyond the status quo of the masses. Men and women of exceptional achievement have therefore always been those who have rejected the programmed mediocrity of the masses, or who have been rejected and judged by the many. The tribe of many has always viewed the tribe of one as antagonistic to its existence – excellence challenges the old values of mediocrity.

17. *Mishenen xa-ahu senet*

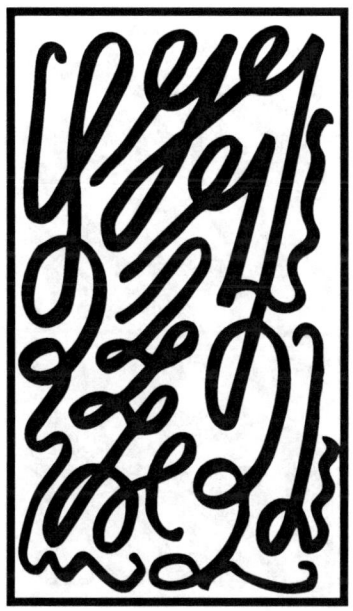

Today's mediocrity should not be judged as less worthy of existing than the excellence of the few wayshowers of humanity. Today's excellence will be tomorrow's mediocrity, just as today's mediocrity was yesterday's excellence. The existing level of the masses' expression provides the firm foundation from which the extraordinary flight of the few can begin the stable change of the many.

18. Erksavu plihabasat nanun

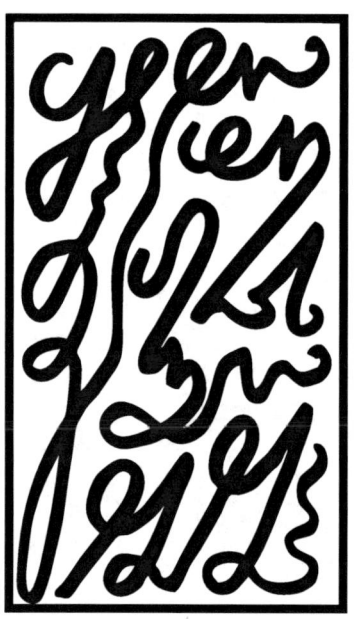

Pride comes from affirming our validity by the role we play. Those who strive to maintain the old value systems of the many, pride themselves in being the pillars of society. Those who rise beyond existing paradigms, pride themselves in being system busters and harbingers of positive change. In the same way, the stability of the floor is needed in order to provide the necessary resistance for your feet to walk, so all roles work together in equal validity to express infinite being into finite expression.

19. Kitra bisheneng nanu hashung

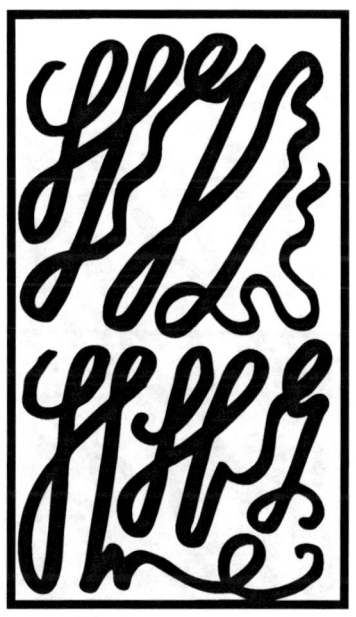

The moral certitude with which we defend our way as the most valid, stems from the mistaken belief that existence needs to be justified. One thread in the intricate pattern of a spider web is not more necessary than another. Each thread of the web of expressed life is part of the perfection of the design. The validity of each life form lies in its beingness as much as in its doingness – that unique response to life that comes from that individual's specific perspective.

20. Plabashing petrenus harashanun

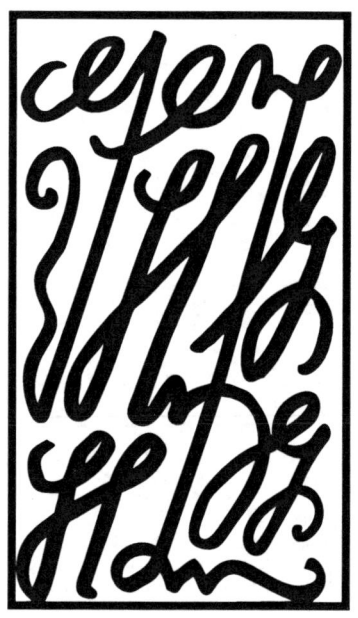

The next step of the Eternal Dance of existence is prompted by either positive (constructive) promptings of the heart, or negative (destructive) situations. When we do not express that which prompts us within, we encounter roadblocks without, on the journey of life. Realizing that as an individual, or a society, we create the perpetrators in our life and then condemn them, we can begin to understand that punitive justice will simply produce more criminals. Infinite existence choreographs its own expression. We either participate with grace, or through being coerced by circumstances.

21. *Eksunim peleshin prekprahun*

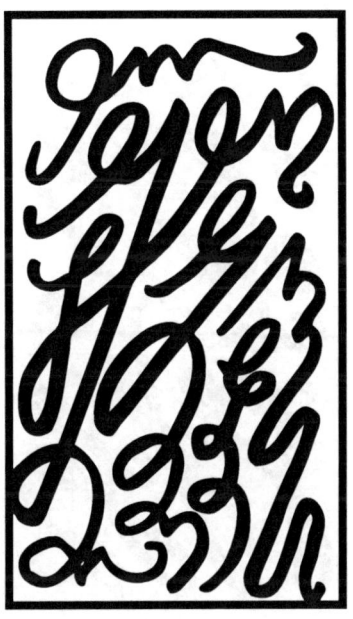

The degree to which we can master space and time, depends very much on how unencumbered we are by associations and memories and programs of yesterday. The one who lives with full awareness of the newness of the moment, sets in motion a tide of opportunities he cannot imagine. To step free from the influence of the past, allows it to fluidly change from the present. In return, the past now enhances the present's potential, and linear time begins to close down on itself. Exponential change becomes available to us, creating more effortless accomplishment.

22. Akvavresba ashaning nesunat

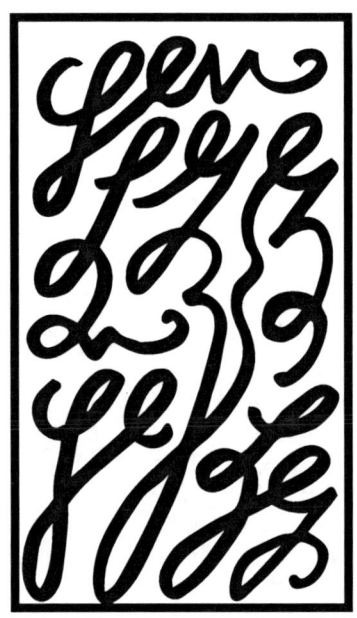

Our identities were meant to be mere roles we can vary at will, the way a child dresses up in play. To identify with our deeds and choices of the past, is to incarcerate ourselves within our limited vision of yesterday. Our associations with the past, keep both ourselves and the past from changing. Look at the identities you have allowed yourself to assume with as much soberness as possible, and know they are but momentary roles. Fear may follow when we let these familiar shelters go, but fear heralds the transcendence of all old paradigms. Move through the fear with understanding.

23. Kelenes nusavi enes eresta

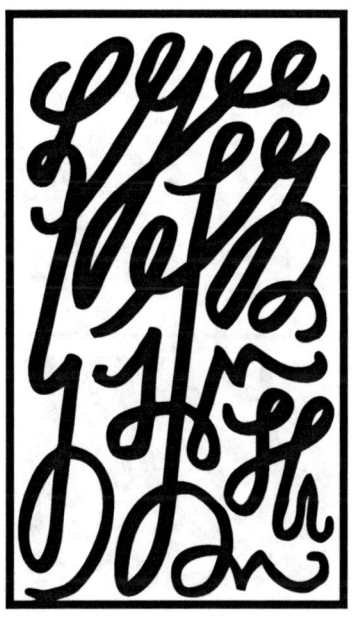

To a tightrope walker in the middle of his journey across his rope, all 100 steps he took before to get to this point do not matter. Only his next step is of concern to him. All the pride or shame connected with previous choices is meaningless. All previous steps have brought us to this moment and it is here where absolute clarity awaits. Full awareness must therefore be given to our next step – in this moment.

24. Habaret yong nate satahay

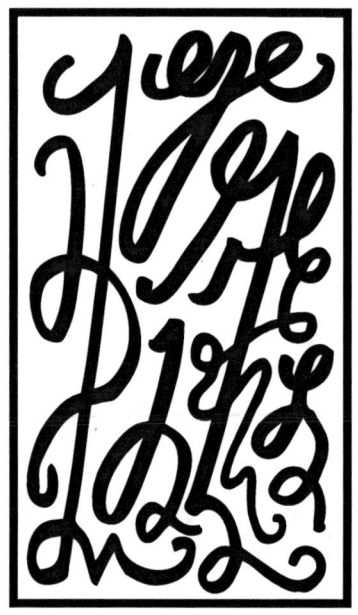

We become what we fight against, just as surely as the tar sticks to the one who works in the tar pit. What you deny the right to exist, will follow you till the ends of the Earth in order to face you through your experiences. What you reject will challenge you again and again, until you acknowledge its right to exist through including it by means of empathic understanding.

25. *Xianung zingtanay pareshet vinas*

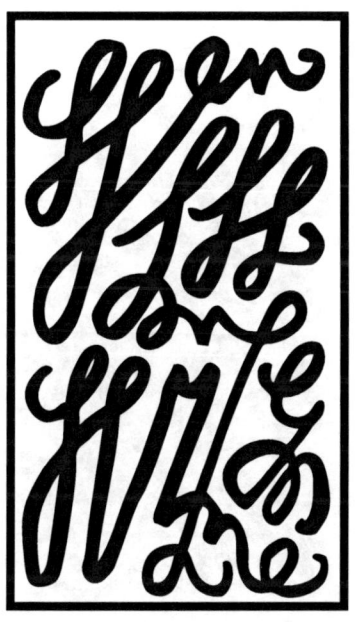

To shift beyond world beliefs seems like an insurmountable task when one considers that you are trying to break free from the matrix kept in place by trillions of people. The matrix is affirmed every time someone lives it, until it seems as thick as concrete. The matrix kept in place by the many, can be shattered by the one when he realizes that it is unreal, and steadfastly rejects it as his reality.

26. Sa-unun tavay akra binasung

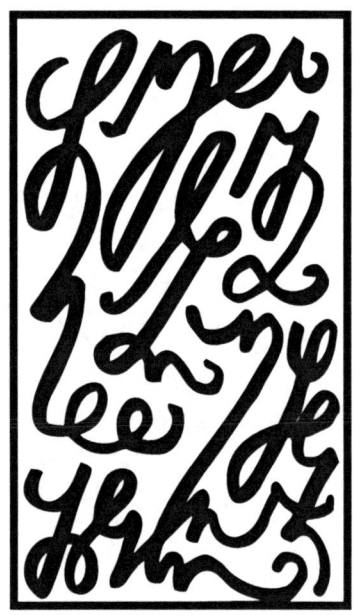

To live beyond world beliefs requires a different perspective that sees beyond their limitation. It is like creating a peephole in the wall of a massive dam. Even though the wall is much bigger than the hole in the wall, the hole will eventually allow the pressure of the water to break down the whole dam. With determination, keep the perspective that sees into a new reality.

27. *Kese hut natava vi-aravi*

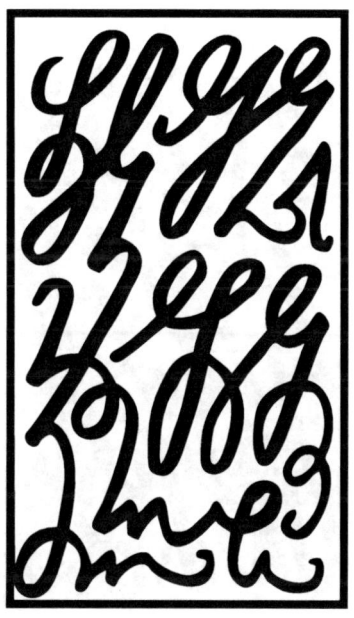

For eons, those who have wanted to transcend the reality of the masses, have kept others of similar vision around them to help affirm the new paradigm. They have formed mystery schools, temples and ashrams to help keep the world and its lower paradigm out. But what was resisted always forced its way in, one way or another. What was chosen as a new viewpoint to live by, was no more valid than the viewpoint of another. It was still the product of selective vision that rejected one paradigm over another.

28. Aknung selhat ubasetvi

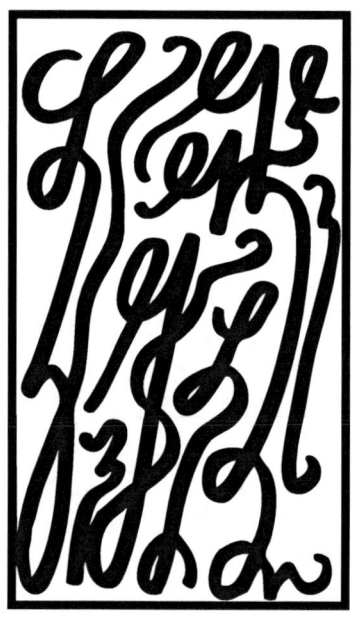

The one who wishes to live free from belief systems' imprisonment, can only prevent another set of belief systems from forming by completely releasing the need to know, in favor of the wonderment of experience. This cannot be done by excluding one part of experience in favor of another, but by living from beyond either. To do this we release value judgments and live as a participating spectator, forming anew from the unformed, without the fetters of self-reflection.

29. Krihanung saraset xi-aho nas

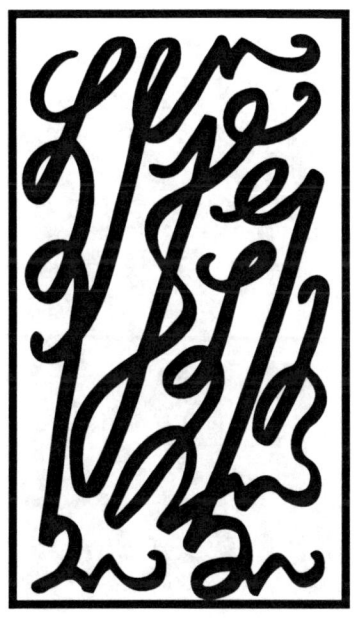

There is an inherent judgment against decay versus rejuvenation. The desire to maintain youthfulness is wrapped in spiritual terms and seen as an indicator of a surrendered life. Age is seen in some cultures as an indicator of wisdom, or accumulated knowledge. Beyond either age or wisdom lies the exquisite expression of agelessness exploring itself in innocence.

30. Li-anung sebeta plihet

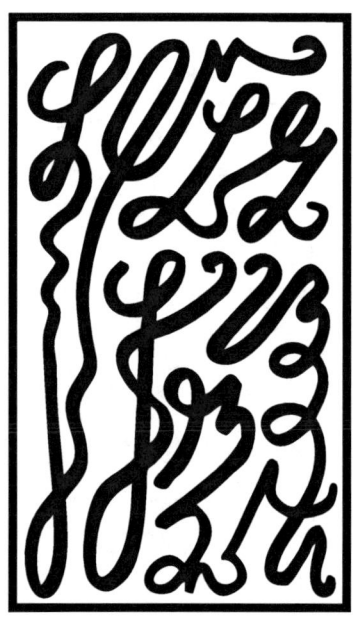

Relationships bind when they are conditional attachments. Examine your interaction with others to see where the relationship is dependent on specific roles and identities that either one is required to play. When the relationship is based on mutual contribution in order to bring about a certain result, it should periodically be examined to make sure that all aspects of your agreement and goal are still valid to you both. Many relationships endure only because of lack of self-sovereignty and fear of change.

31. Tu-avanet sihater plihanu anang

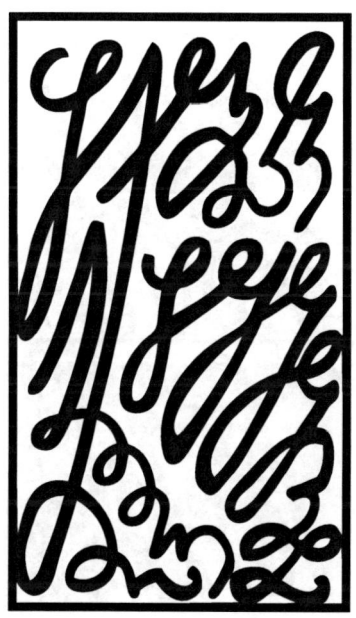

A relationship should be the interaction of mutually contributed elements to produce an unfolding, living work of art. Release with grace that which no longer inspires the poetry in your heart, that the next contributing elements may enter to continue the inspired art of your eternal existence.

32. Keseti anay yihanunang save

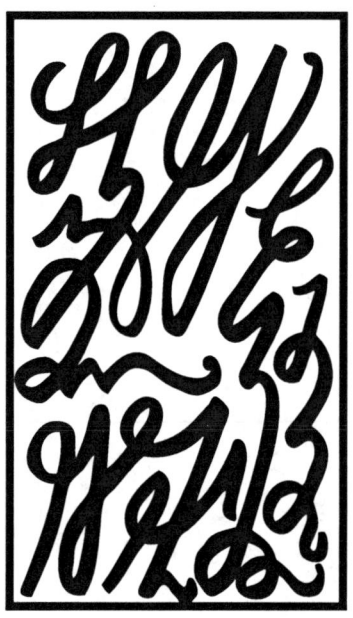

Many cling to relationships because they are afraid of being alone. Togetherness gives the opportunity to examine the details of the unique poetic expression of yourself within the mirror of another. Aloneness allows you to find the eternal perspective within the vastness of your being. Do not neglect the gifts of either, by emphasizing only one or the other.

33. Parasetanut vishenung xian anani

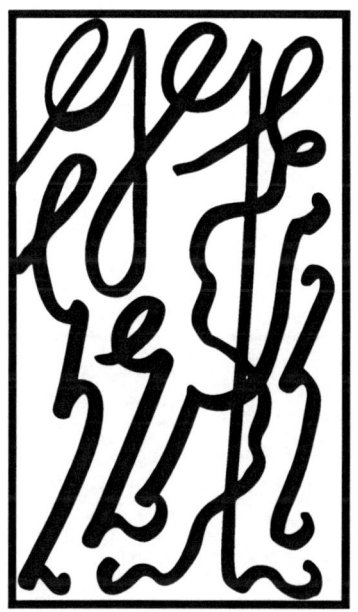

Aging is often manifested as a relief from having to constantly give, be productive, be responsible. By manifesting a second childhood through the helplessness of age, the person finally feels entitled to receive. To combat this powerless way of trying to manipulate life, it is necessary to:

- Cultivate generosity and contribution in the early years of childhood, at whatever level the child is able to give.
- To live in a way that inspires us, taking time to know and express the nuances of our heart.
- To guard against any areas in which we abandon self-expression, and to take drastic steps to reestablish full expression. It is from the hollow life of self-abandonment, that we live only to serve others and other causes. The pain of alienation from the

authentic expression of ourselves is alleviated by the formation of addictions.

- It is necessary for the elderly to contribute in ways that bring them satisfaction. Avoid at all costs allowing the unacceptable because of age, or you will find yourself being manipulated by it.

34. Kasha-anung selhat usa versanun

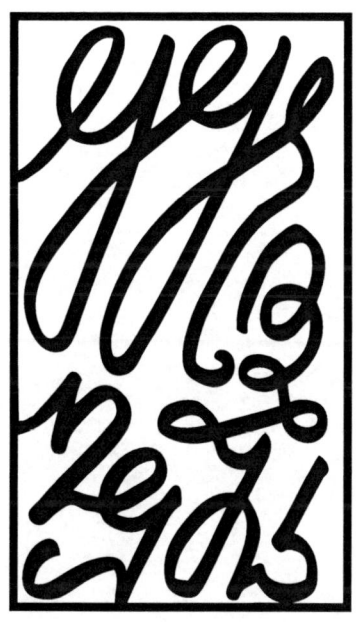

Do not fight against, nor be intimidated by the illusions of life. They are but the tools you wield to create the artistry of expression of your being. As you embrace them as part of your dance, learning from them about your being's own aspects, you will eventually learn how to express the magnificence of your being without the use of imagined tools.

The Breathing Techniques
of the Twelve Breaths of Proxy

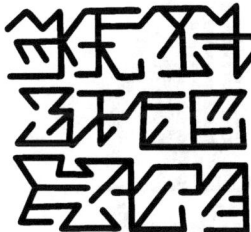 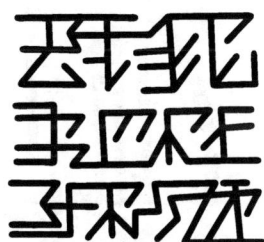

Radiation obtained from seafood and sea plants, electrical devices, some water sources and more, accumulate in women's mammary glands and in men's prostate glands. These breaths are designed to purify these and other centers. Increase water intake when doing these exercises.

1. Shez-su-anan
The Breath to Cleanse the Valves of the Body

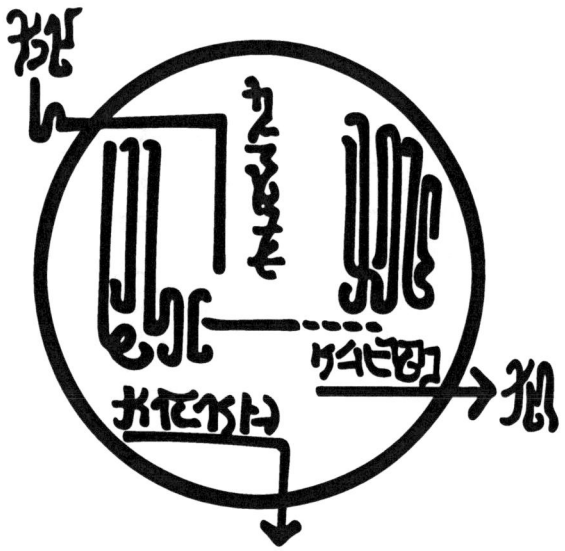

Posture:
- Sit on the floor with your spine straight and the soles of your feet together. Start with your head erect, chin level to the floor.
- Place the two index fingers on either side of the bridge of the nose. The thumbs are pressing on the points ¾ of an inch from the outer corners of the eyes. These points are about the length of the top digit of your thumb out from the eyes, just within the soft part of the temple.
- The other fingers are relaxed and the elbows are out to the side.

The Breath:
- Keep the spine straight as you breathe in deeply while maintaining firm pressure on the bridge of the nose.
- Breathe out through the mouth with short, staccato puffs of air. With each puff of breath, relax the back and head forward in

an arc. The arching of the back will be done in sporadic, jerky movement.

- The arms and hands remain in the same position.
- Straighten the spine again on the next deep in-breath.
- There will be a total of 12 in-and out-breaths.

Note: All 12 Breaths of Proxy are repeated 12 times each.

2. Baranang-surat

The Breath to Cleanse the Lymph Terminals

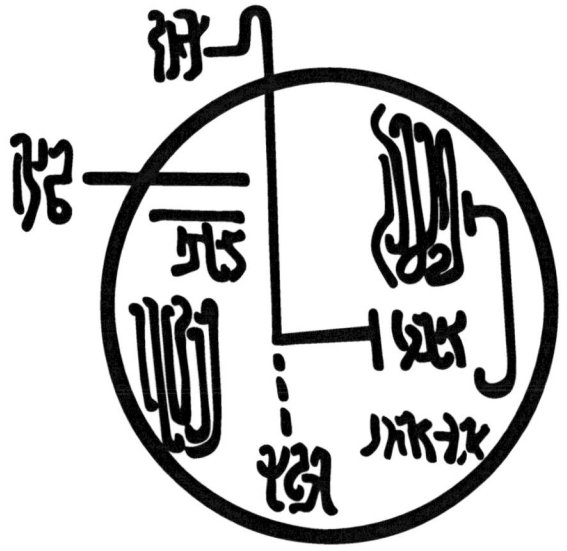

Posture:

- Sit with your spine straight and the soles of your feet together.
- Rest your hands on your thighs, with palms facing upwards and fingers relaxed.
- Start with your chin level to the floor.
- Prior to starting the breath, be sure to locate the two tapping points about the width of 3 fingers below the center of the collarbone. These are the two main lymph terminals.

The Breath:

- Inhale deeply and as you do, move the head as far back as is comfortable. Keep your jaw relaxed and your mouth slightly open on the in-breath. Hold the breath for as long as possible while, with three middle fingers of each hand, tapping firmly on the two lymph terminals.

- On the forceful out-breath, lower your head onto your chest and drop your hands.
- Repeat for a total of 12 in- and out-breaths.

Note: The lymph terminals are usually sensitive to pressure and can sometimes be felt as little nodes beneath the skin.

The Two Main Lymph Terminals Below The Collar Bones

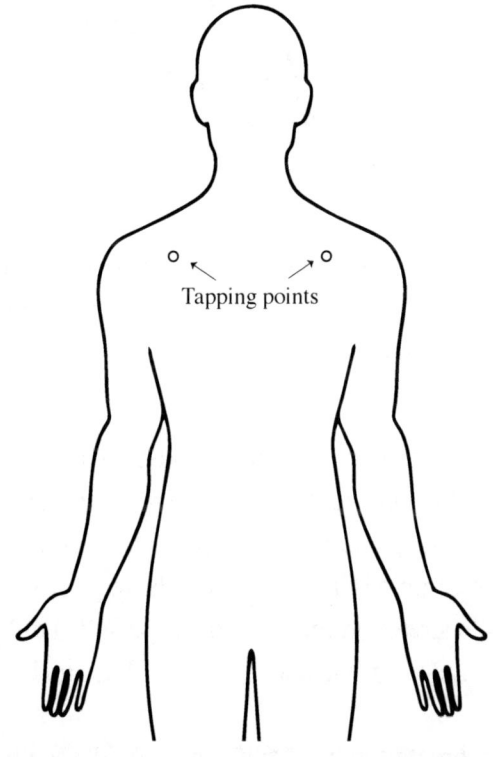

Tapping points

3. Bishete-nanusang
The Breath to Cleanse the Muscles between the Ribs

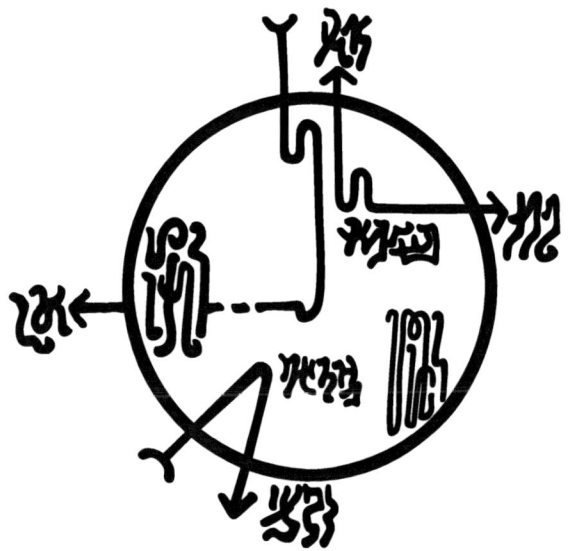

Posture:
- Sit with your spine straight and legs crossed. Your hands will be lying loosely on your thighs, palms up. Your head is facing forward with your chin level to the floor.

The Breath:
- Take a long, smooth in-breath (filling the lungs as full as possible), while moving the hands outward in an arc until they are fully extended in a V-shape above your head. The final position of the arms should resemble wings extended above your shoulders.
- Create a gentle stretch in the chest muscles and shoulders by keeping the arms as far back as possible. Hold the breath for 5 seconds.
- During the in-breath the head and eyes should rise upwards as far as they can comfortably go (like looking up towards the heavens).

- On the out-breath (long and smooth), move the arms down in an arc and back onto the lap, palms up. The head and eyes return to the original position looking straight ahead, chin level to the floor.
- When all the breath has been released, wait 5 seconds before starting the next in-breath.
- Repeat for a total of 12 in- and out-breaths.

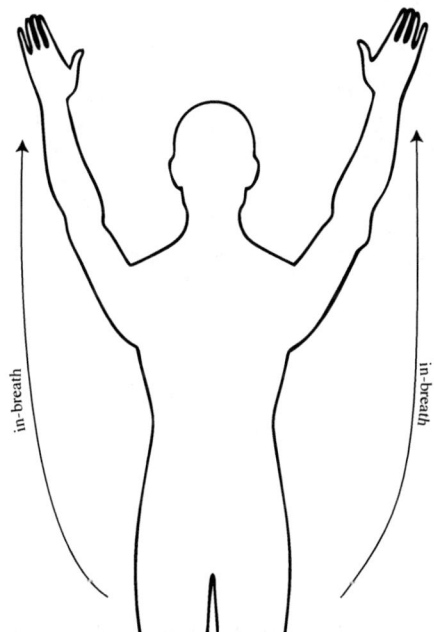

As you raise your arms, raise your head and eyes upwards, looking towards the heavens.

On the out-breath, sweep your arms downwards in an arc, returning your hands to your thighs, with palms facing upwards.

4. Barushang-xianing
The Breath to Cleanse the Membranes of the Lungs

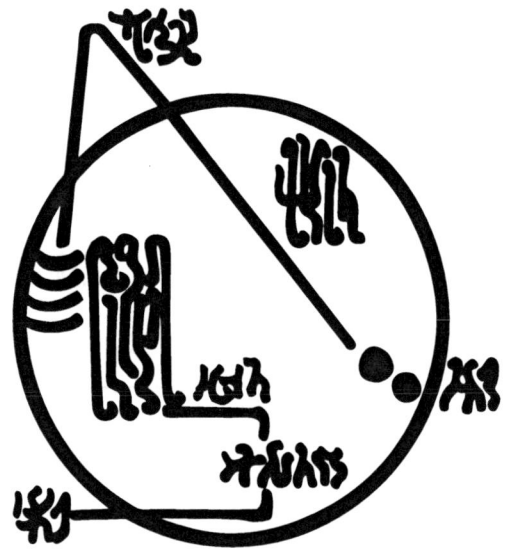

Posture:
- While in a seated position, your spine is straight and your legs are crossed. Your head is facing forward, chin level to the floor.
- Your hands remain lying in a relaxed position on your thighs (palms up) during the in- and out-breaths.

The Breath:
- During the in-breath, imagine your sternum and ribcage being pulled directly forward as though a string were attached to your breastbone. Fill the lungs as full as possible.
- The forward movement of the chest should be kept as isolated as possible. Try not to lean forward from the hips but instead, move only the ribcage while keeping the rest of the body as still as possible.

- The out-breath is released in short staccato bursts of air as the ribcage moves back as far as possible in short, jerking movements.
- Drop the head onto the chest with the same jerking movements during the out-breath.
- With the next in-breath, the head will move smoothly back to its upright position.
- Repeat for a total of 12 in- and out-breaths.

5. *Vivesak-urutu*
The Breath to Cleanse the Diaphragm

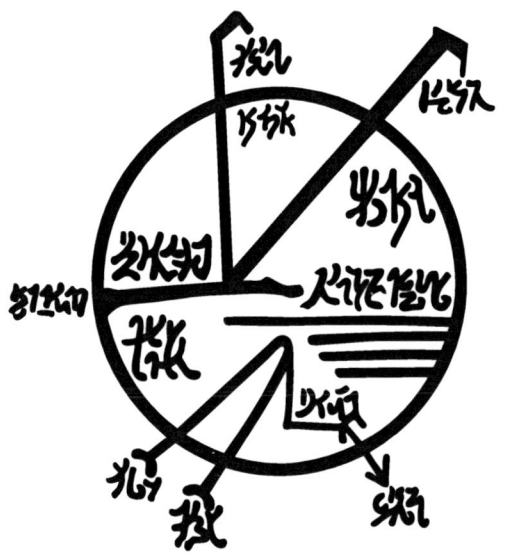

Posture:

- Sit with your feet together, spine and head straight, chin level to the floor and your hands firmly grasping your knees.
- Looking forward, the head position remains the same throughout this breath.

The Breath:

- During the in- and out-breath, the only change in the body position is the isolated movement of the rib cage. Keep the rest of the body as still as possible.
- The rib cage will be moving in a vertical circle, like the water wheel of a watermill. The isolated movement of the rib cage begins with the rib cage moving back as far as possible and then arcing it upwards on the in-breath. The in-breath is done as you complete the back half of the circular movement of the rib cage.

- On the out-breath, move your chest forward and downwards in a arc, completing the front half of the circular movement.
- Repeat for a total of 12 in- and out-breaths.

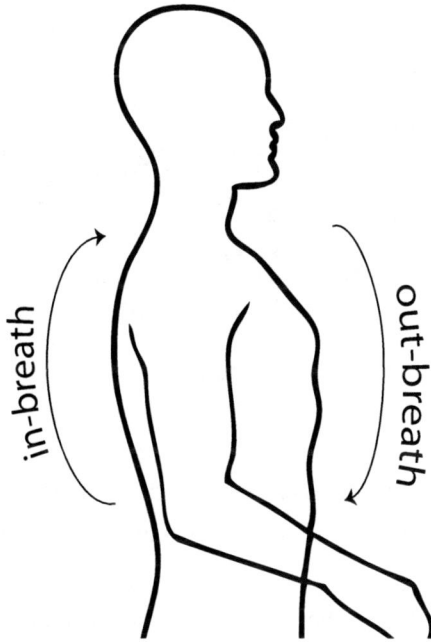

6. Shihet-anunasang
The Breath to Cleanse the Band of Internal Organs Below the Rib Cage

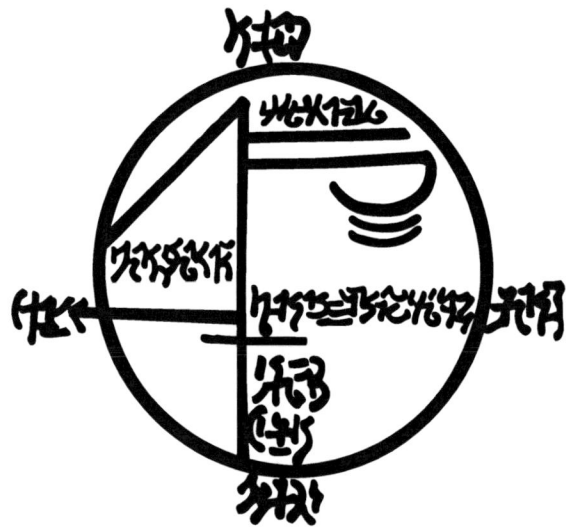

Posture:
- This breath is exactly the same as Breath 5 in all ways, except that the circular movements of the rib cage move in the opposite direction.
- Sit with your feet together, spine and head straight and your hands firmly grasping the knees.
- The position of the head, with the chin level to the floor, remains the same throughout this breath.

The Breath:
- Keeping the rest of the body as still as possible, move the rib cage in a vertical circular movement. Begin by pushing the rib cage as far forward as possible, then arcing it upwards on the in-breath, completing the front half of the circular movement of the rib cage.

- On the out-breath, move the chest back and down while you breathe out all the air from your lungs, completing the back half of the circular movement.
- Repeat for a total of 12 in- and out-breaths.

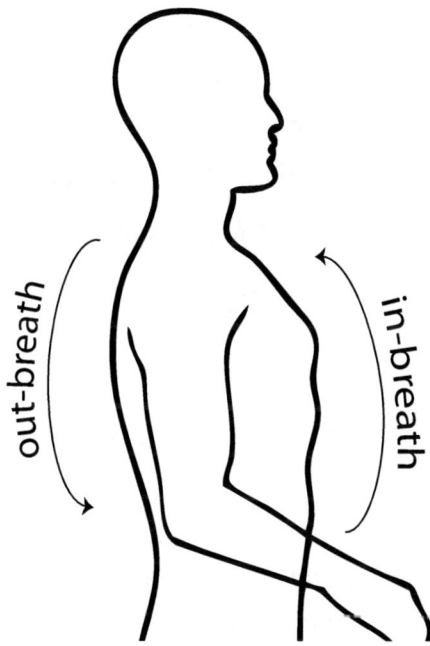

7. Eknetnut-zhinavanay
The Breath to Cleanse the Gastrointestinal Tract

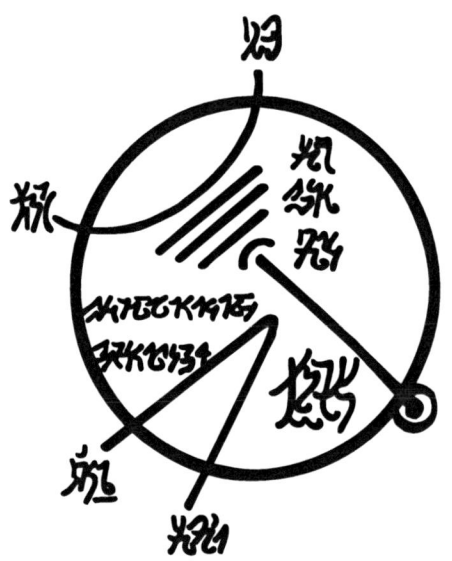

Posture:

- Lie flat on your back, arms and hands lying in a relaxed position by your side.

The Breath:

- During this breath, the abdomen will be moving in a circular pattern while the rest of the body remains as still and relaxed as possible. There will be slight movements in the chest caused by the rolling of the stomach.
- On the in-breath, make the abdominal area as hollow as possible. Beginning in the lower abdomen, make an arc of contraction by drawing the stomach down towards the spine and rolling it up towards the diaphragm. This movement create the lower half of the circular pattern.

- As you breathe out, roll the abdomen upwards and then down in an arc that extends from the diaphragm to the bottom of the abdomen. On the out-breath, the upper half of the circular pattern is created.
- Repeat the in-and out-breaths 12 times while smoothly rolling the belly in a circle. Practice will help make this movement easier.

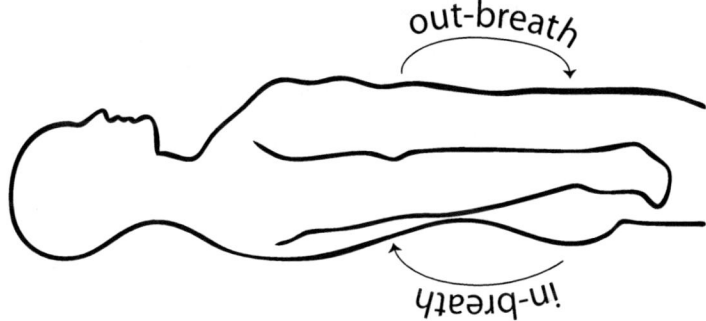

8. Pruhas-sanung

The Breath that Clears the Naval – the Source of Neediness

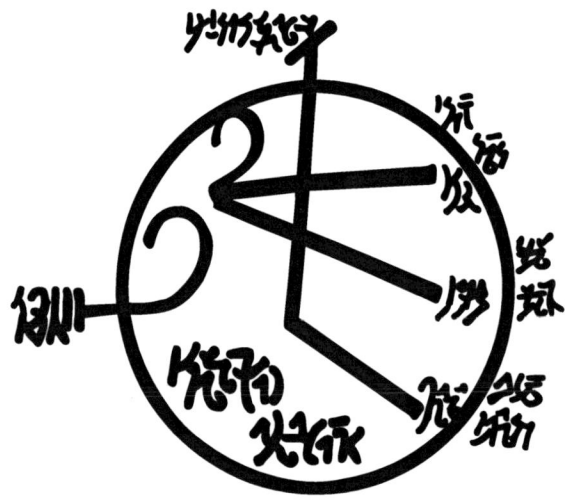

Posture:

- Lie flat on your back, hands and arms relaxed by your side.
- Bend your knees by drawing your feet closer to your body. The feet will be about shoulder-width apart.

The Breath:

- With a long, deep breath – draw in as much air as you can into the lungs.
- The out-breath is a short burst of breath that you imagine coming out of the navel like a 'pop,' as though a cork has been removed.
- As the out-breath is released, the hips will rise slightly off the ground. A slight, rapid extension of the stomach during the out-breath may assist in moving the energy.
- Repeat for a total of 12 in- and out-breaths.

9. Peshanang-Zhihani
The Breath to Clear the Reproductive System

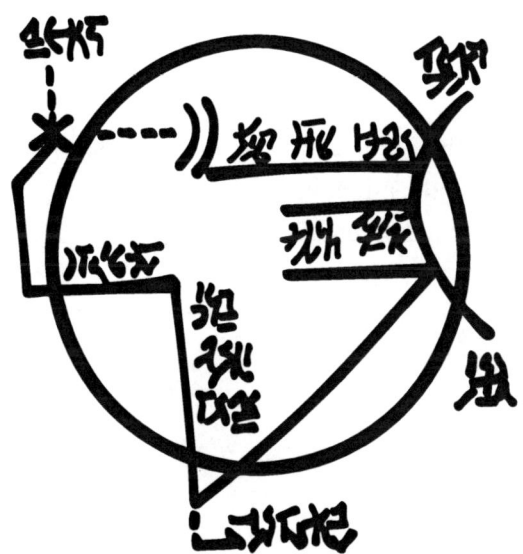

Posture:

- Lie flat on your back, hands and arms relaxed by your side.
- Bend your knees by drawing your feet closer to your body. The feet will be about shoulder-width apart. During this breath, your hips will be raised off the floor.

The Breath:

- For the first 6 repetitions of the in-and out-breaths, the hips will draw a figure 8 through the air starting with the left hip.
- Starting on the in-breath, move the left hip down and circle it upwards.
- As you breathe out, move the right hip down and then upwards.
- Every time you draw the left part of the figure 8, you will be breathing in. When creating the right side of the vertical figure 8, you will be breathing out.

- When you have completed your in-breath for the 6th time, hold the hip movement still (at the middle-point) to do the out-breath.

Breaths 7 – 12 are the reverse of Breaths 1 – 6.
- On the 7th in-breath, start with the right hip and move it down and circle it upwards.
- As you transition to the out-breath, move the left hip down and circle back up to the midpoint.
- Continue for the next 5 breaths.

10. Keena-nay-atyang

The Clearing of the Root Chakra and Buttock Muscles

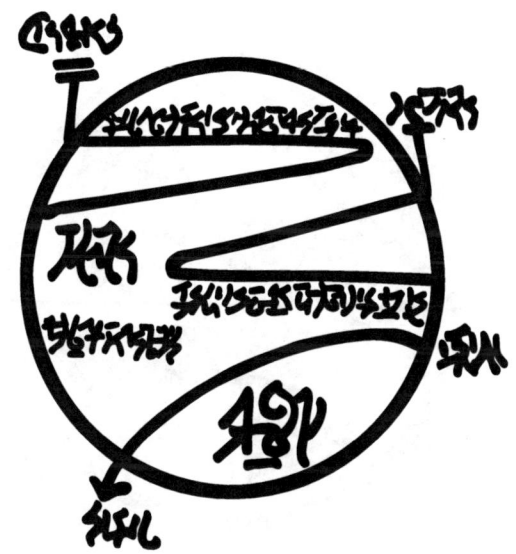

Posture:

- Lie flat on your back, hands and arms relaxed by your side.
- Bend your knees by drawing the feet closer to your body. The feet will be about shoulder-width apart.

The Breath:

- The in-breath is slow and deep. As you breathe in, raise the hips and tighten the buttock muscles.
- Hold the breath for about 5 seconds, keeping the buttocks tight and raised.
- Release the breath rapidly and with some force, as you drop the hips back down to the floor, releasing all tension.
- Repeat for a total of 12 in- and out-breaths.

11. Aze-vanastan
The Breath to Clear the Hip Joints and Thighs

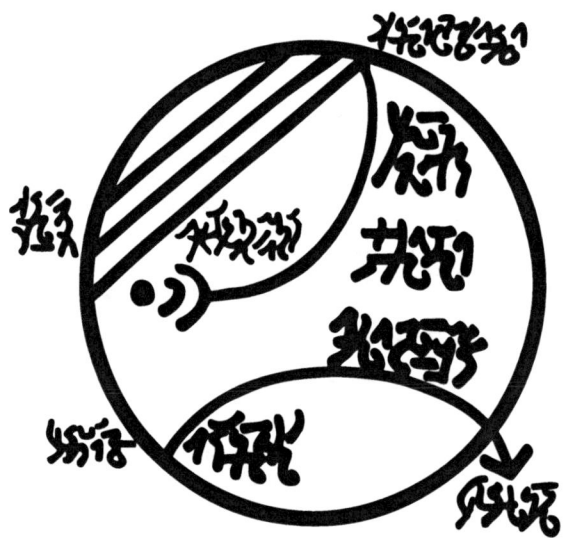

Posture:
- Lie flat on your back, hands and arms relaxed by your side.
- Bend your knees by drawing your feet closer to your body and place the feet together so that they are touching each other.
- The hips are raised above the floor for the duration of this Breath.

The Breath:
- During the in- and out-breaths, the hips will move up and down slightly, like a gentle pulse. They will move up with the in-breath and down with the out-breath, without touching the ground for the remainder of this Breath.
- Breathe in, moving the knees apart, while keeping the feet together and raise the hips slightly.
- Breathe out while moving the knees together and lowering the hips slightly.

- The movements and breaths are smooth and resemble the pulsating movements of the wings of a resting butterfly.
- Repeat for a total of 12 in- and out-breaths.

12. Chabaruk-mishangve
The Breath to Release Heavy Metals from the Bloodstream

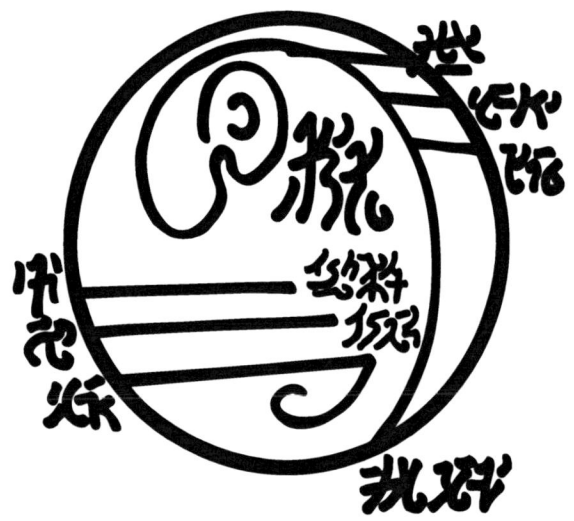

Posture:

* Lie flat on your back, legs and arms straight and relaxed. Your eyes remain closed for the duration of this Breath.

The Breath:

* Breathe in deeply and while holding your breath for as long as possible, shake the body from head to toes without changing position. This is done by shaking various muscle groups, such as the thighs, calves and buttocks for instance.
* Breathe out in a long sigh and completely relax the body.
* Repeat for a total of 12 in- and out-breaths.

Note: The shaking should create small enough movements that you do not injure your neck or other muscles.

Closing

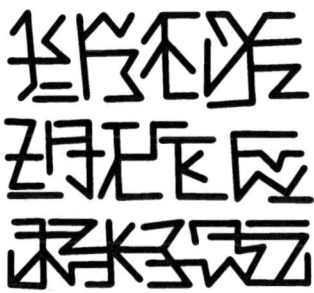

We are living in exciting times full of wonder and magic, and the greatest of opportunities to profoundly and beneficially impact global life.

The human race is being evolved into a more highly developed state of being – one in which illness is a mere reminder of unexpressed portions of ourselves. These reminders become more painless and transient as we learn to acknowledge and respond to them as masters of the quality of our journey. As the few take responsibility for the cleansing of the bloodstream by purifying the emotions (and thereby cleansing the environment), they become unaffected by radiation. As with all illusions that appear to affect us, we use the tools of power to eliminate them.

It can be asked that if we create our realities by what we emphasize and focus on, will engaging with illusion not ultimately enforce its presence? The answer to the seeming contradiction of getting rid of some illusion (like radiation), even though we know it does not exist, lies in the following realizations:

- Our focus should not be on the radiation as we do the breaths, but on the eternal newness of our being.

- As we hold the vision of our indestructible and timeless existence, while doing the breathing techniques on behalf of the many, we are able to lessen the effects of the illusion for them as well.
- Any pollution or disease is a reminder to allow the unexpressed portions of our being to come forth. We engage with these signals as though they are real just long enough to ascertain the next step in the dance of life. We then shift our focus to the new expression we have awakened, on our never-ending cosmic dance.
- In the aftermath of the atomic bomb of Hiroshima, it was discovered that 3 people who had been near the blast, were completely unaffected by the radiation. In subsequent studies, certain commonalities in their diets (like ginseng) were discovered, but others who perished had used them too. The hidden truth behind this miracle is that they had become sovereign in the knowledge that their being has always existed and was completely unable to be affected by the world as a mirrored reflection around them.

Enhancing the Nutritional Frequency of Food

Stimulating the Nutritional Frequency of Food

Method

Create a stack of the following wheels:

- At the bottom place *The Clock of Spirit from the Hidden Realms.*

- Next place *The Lemurian Clock of the Depth of Living.*

- Then using the 3 *Wheels to Stimulate the Nutritional Frequencies of Food* – place *Wheel 3,* followed by *Wheel 2* and on top place *Wheel 1.*

Place the food on top of the stack of Wheels and Clocks and leave it there for at least 20 minutes. For repeated use you may want to laminate them.

Removing Radiation from Food

To remove radiation from food, place a 6th Wheel – *The Clock of Light* – on the bottom of the stack below *The Clock of Spirit from the Hidden Realms.* This is the only wheel to work on the physical level. The use of this wheel is especially recommended for seafood and sea vegetables.

The Clock of Spirit from the Hidden Realms

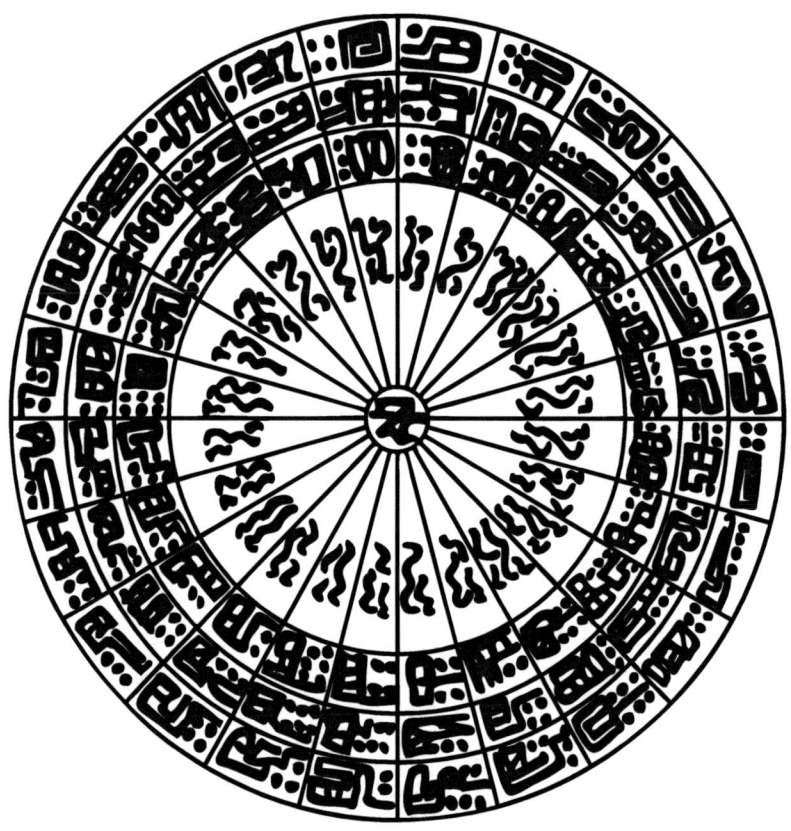

The Lemurian Clock of the Depth of Living

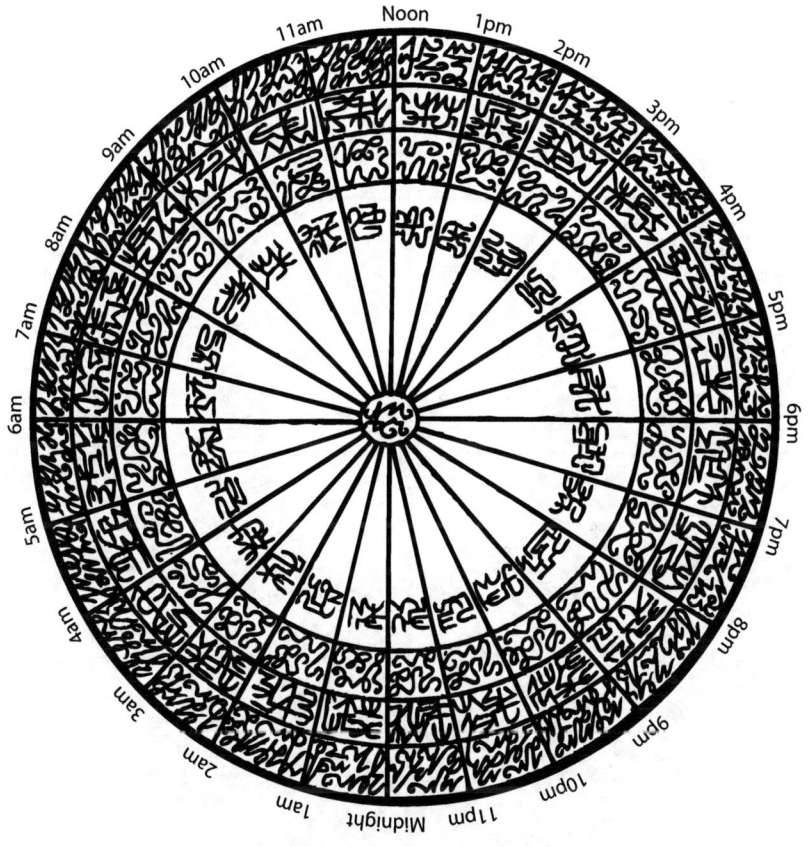

Vaareska Unespa Heresvi Bareshtu
Indivisible Oneness is all that Exists

Wheel 3
To Stimulate the Nutritional Frequency of Food

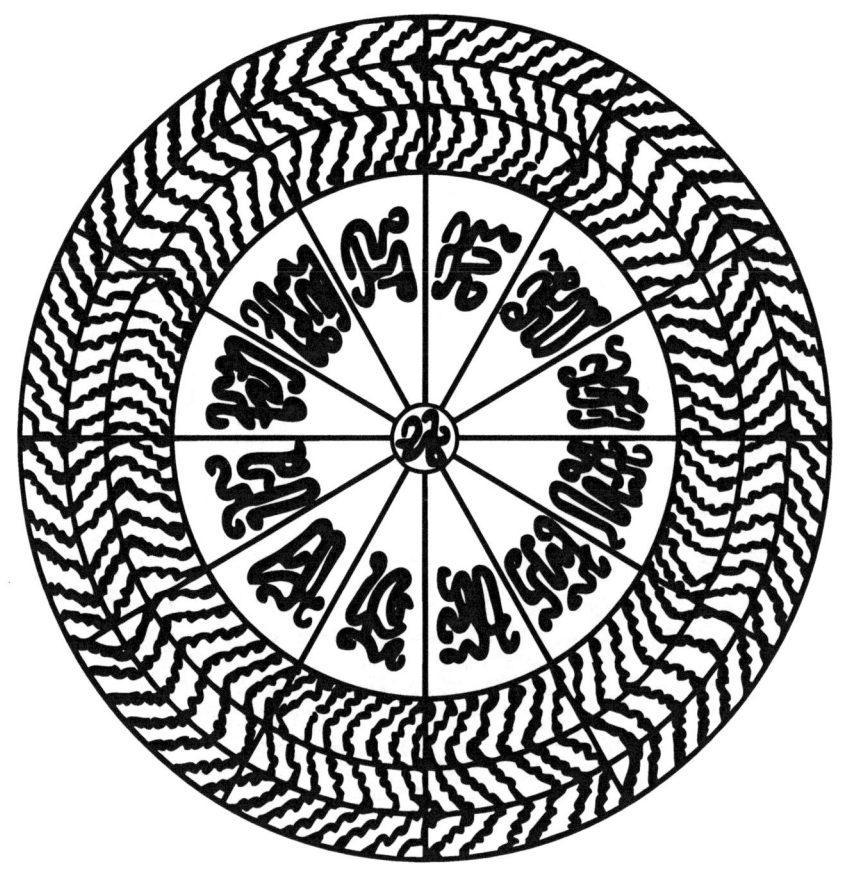

Wheel 2
To Stimulate the Nutritional Frequency of Food

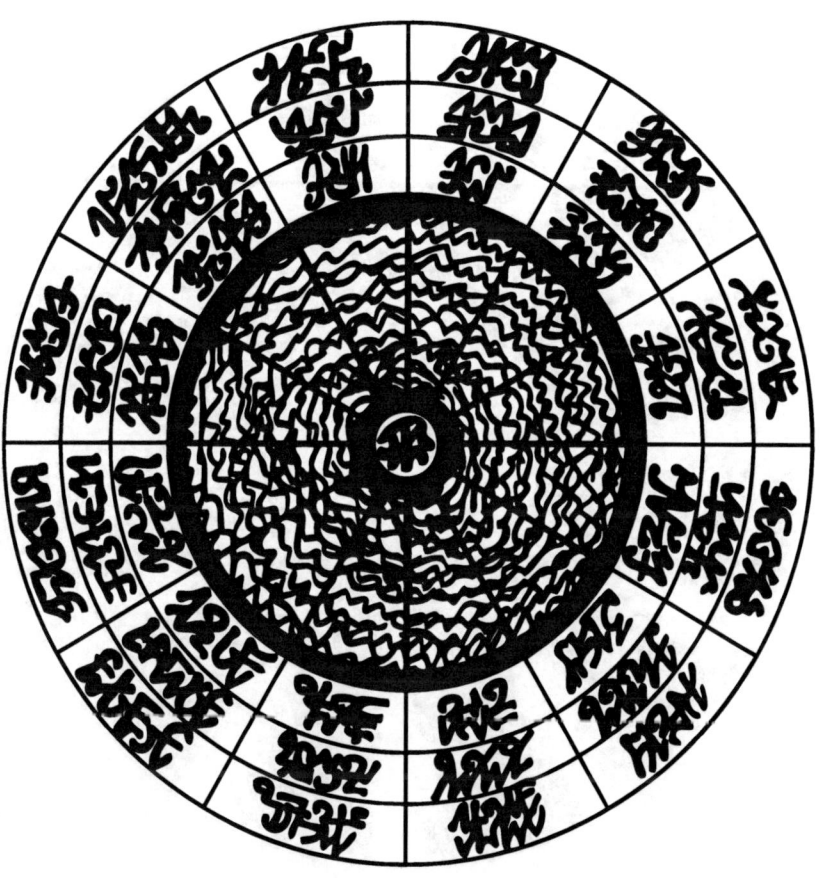

Wheel 1

To Stimulate the Nutritional Frequency of Food

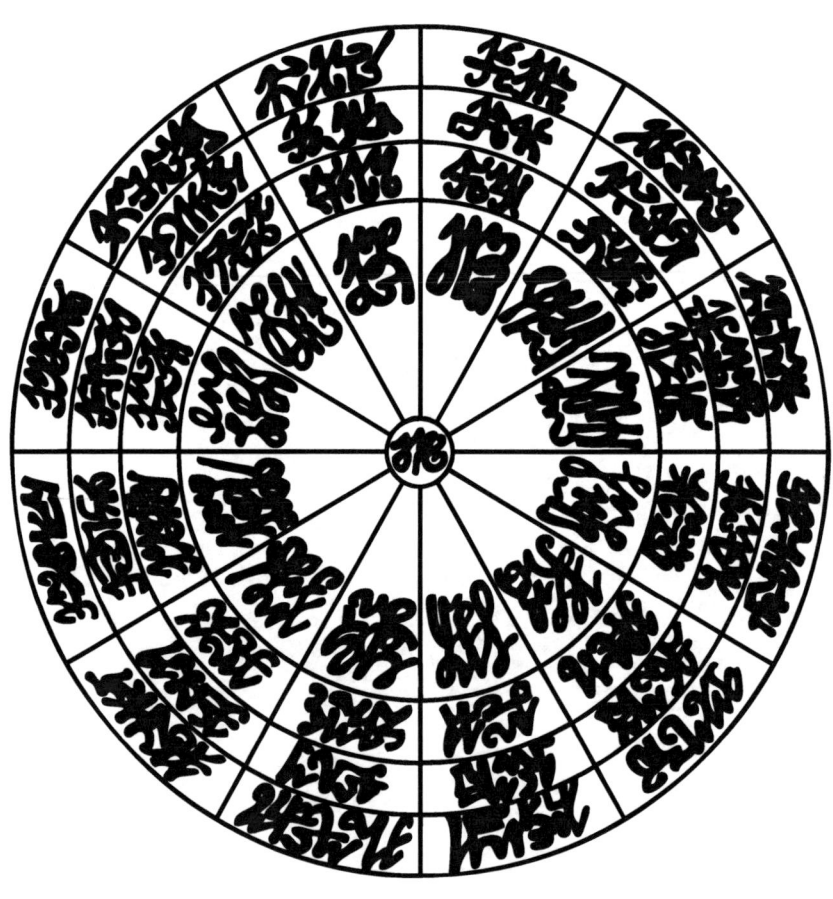

The Clock of Light

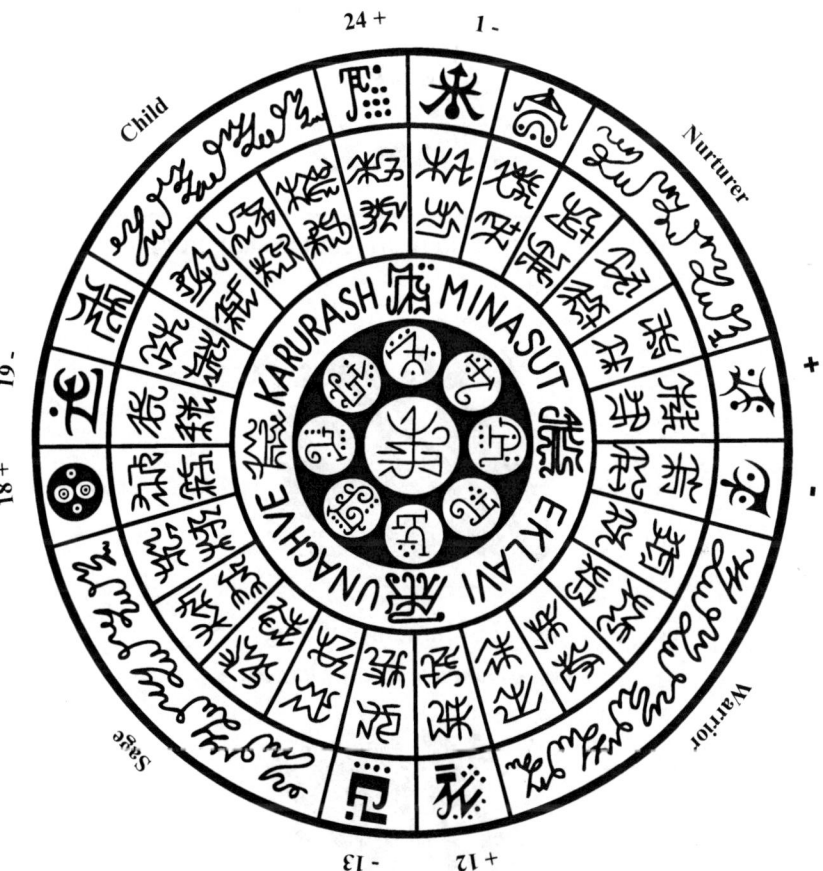

Sigils for the Purification of Linear Time

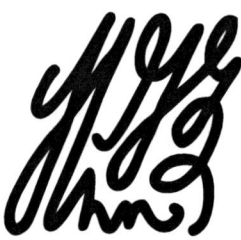

For the removal of empowerment through proximity.

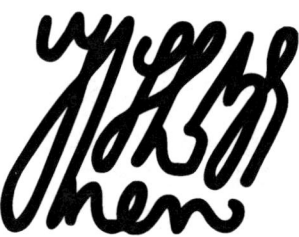

For the removal of influence through arrogance
due to a sense of entitlement.

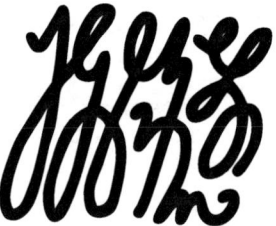

For the dissolving of old hierarchies and their
cosmic influences and tyrannies.

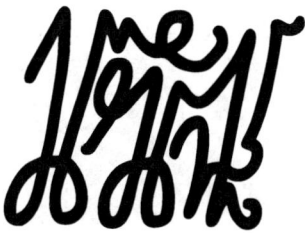

For the dissolving of old, unholy alliances of
control and personal aggrandizement.

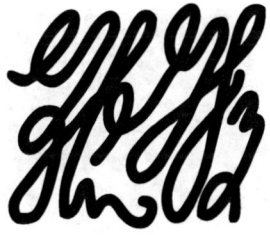

For the removal of hierarchies based
on sequences of creation.

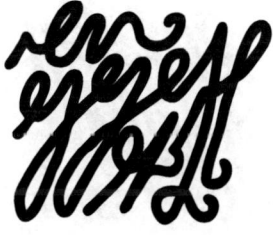

For the removal of governments designed to undermine, obscure
and disconnect life forms from Source.

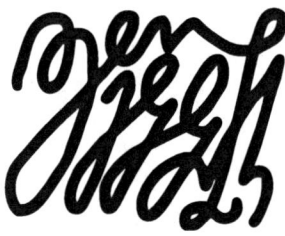

For the removal of future schemes and
strategies to seize control.

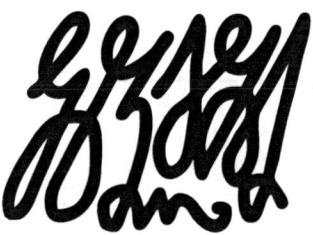

For the removal of the bondage of black magic
to blind and control cosmic beings.

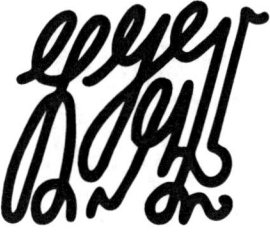

For the removal of all plans and mechanisms to
bring back old stories and dreams of the past.

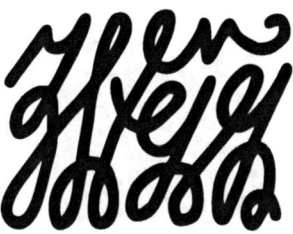

For the removal of brainwashing and all controlling strategies
of fear, greed, pain, protectiveness, anger and guilt.

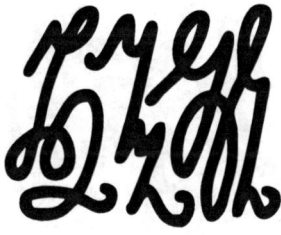

For the removal of the hostile influences
of the super-gods and primary gods.

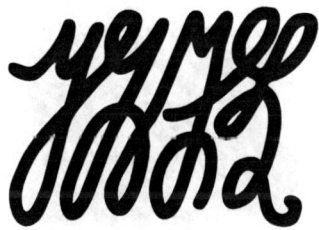

For the removal of the ability to disseminate
untruth about the Source of Existence.

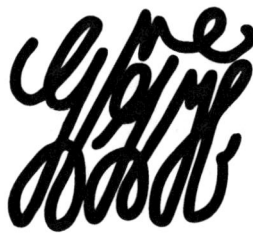

For the removal of the web of existence and the dissolving
of old matrices of all types of subversive control.

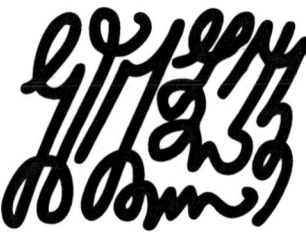

For the reestablishment of the recognition
of the purity of the Infinite.

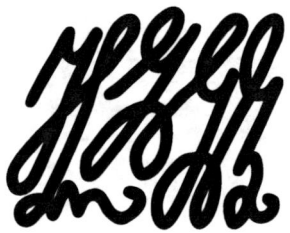

For absolute trust in the benevolence of the expression
of the Infinite Being even when not understood.

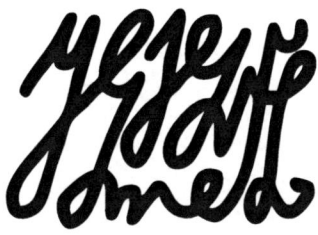

For cooperative expression of the unimpeded
flow and emphasis of Infinite Intent.

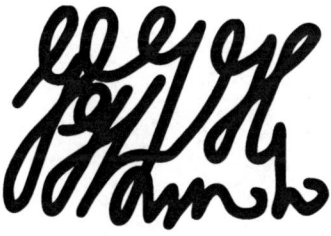

For the replacing of old masculine hierarchal
regimes with power through merit.

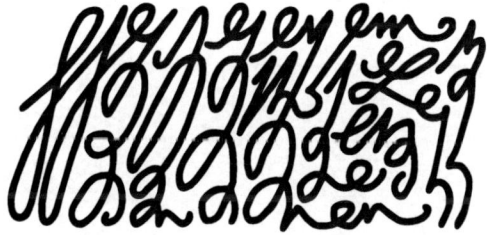

For the advent of the reign of peace and joy of the
Embodiment of the Infinite Being, and the
establishment of inspired dynamic balance.

BOOK THREE

Ma-atma Suhat

The Breaths of Evolved Awareness

Great is the awareness that shall be birthed,
when the full refrain of purity sounds on
Earth.

Ma-atma Suhat

Level I – Sa-huna Satma

The Breaths of Higher Consciousness

The Birth of a Higher Consciousness

An interview with the Seer Almine
by Serge, Canada

Q. What is different now that the Mayan Calendar has declared time to have ended in 2012?
A. There are four primary areas of existence that will be profoundly different. These changes will slowly but surely manifest as alterations to our reality. First, a few will change in the way they experience life, then it will ripple through the lives of the multitudes. It is like the scenario of when water changes to steam – first just a few water molecules escape, then eventually all the water becomes steam.

Q. What is the first area of great change?
A. The ending of linear time means that time no longer goes around and around the disc of individuated life in cycles, called incarnations, like a dog chasing its tail. Cycles of life, death and ascension become a choice rather than a necessity.

Q. What is time's movement now, if it isn't circular anymore, and how will that affect everyday life?
A. It has become exponential rather than following the linear progression of cause and effect. Imagine Infinite Expression being like a calm lake. Every act of a being, functioning from the higher level of consciousness, is like a raindrop falling in the lake. It ripples out, without the lake actually moving, intersecting the ripples of the actions of others. Where the ripples intersect, new potential opens up through the awakening of alchemy. This means that great, positive changes are possible if we are open to them.

Q. What is different in the relationship of cause and effect with this new movement of time?

A. These two opposites become integrated; functioning as one. That means your intentions, thoughts and feelings will manifest almost immediately.

Q. What is the second area of change?

A. A lessening of hardship and opposition as our environment changes from a mirrored reflection to a poetic expression.

Q. Why must it be poetic, rather than any other form of expression?

A. To see the poetry of life even in the suffering of others, helps the few trail-blazers of light who escape the matrix of linear time not to get dragged back by the old reality of the many, but rather through the beauty of their lives, express a new one...

Q. Like becoming a living work of art... How is life in our environment viewed by one who expresses his environment, rather than one who tries to define himself by his environment?

A. I want to quote a poem called "The Artist," written by a 13- year old Native American Cree girl.

The Artist

An unknown journey
My pencil, the paper, and I
A single black line on a background of white
The beginning of alchemy of creation yet unborn
A wolf prowling on a snowy night
His silent howl, piercing the moon.

The images pour from my mind
And the paper comes alive
A window into the depth of my soul

The bold yellow eyes challenging me
In a shaft of moonlight, between dark trees
A black figure pauses to look at me
Soft padded paws buried in the snow, his jaw slightly open
Revealing the long white canines, like icicles

Forever frozen in time
Frozen in time…

Jaylene Manitopyes

Q. Please comment on the poem's insights.
A. The artist looks at her artwork as a window into her own soul. The poem gives the paradigm-shifting feeling that all realities are equally alive and real, because all are the expression of the artist, who sees herself in her work. The work sees itself in her. Boundaries between real and unreal, inner and outer, become blurred.

Q. How do we achieve this awareness?
A. By releasing the need for self-reflection; living unselfconsciously like a child. Also by releasing resistance to life through surrendered trust.

Q. What is the third area of change?
A. Cosmic life has become like a resurrected being. Soul and body have blended into one; death and life's alternating cycles have become optional.

Q. Has this already begun?
A. Yes. The soul level of cosmic life, a parallel reality, has blended with ours. Many strange beings have entered our hidden realms that have not been encountered before. I received the *Wheel of Combined Realities* from the angels, showing the alchemical blending of the high angelic realms with physical life.

Q. What is the fourth area of change?
A. The purification of old impressions (akashic imprints) that have created karma. They have lingered like ghosts, calling us back again and again to relive them.

Q. Is this what has caused the cycles of incarnation?
A. Yes, in large part.

Q. How will the purification occur?

A. Through the restoration of lost tones, or frequencies of purity. We have had only 96 active tones of purity, each represented by an angelic order, but there are 144.

Q. Has this been restored, and does this mean that individual karma can also be erased for those who live this higher life?

A. Yes, to both questions. *The Wheel of Perpetual Regeneration through Trust in Self-Sovereignty* contains the sigils (glyphs) representing the 144 Tones of Purity.

Thank you for sharing so much information with us.

The Seer's Wisdom –
The Way of Higher Consciousness

Abundance does not flow from actions alone.
In silent receptivity, await life's generosity.

The Seer's Wisdom

Q. Tell us Master, that we may know, does the poet or the farmer the most consciousness show? Who contributes the most, the farmer who sows the golden grain or the poet's words of joyful refrains?
A. The poet who with his parchment toils, the farmer who writes his poem in the furrowed soil, both are living works of art. Both hear the Infinite's song in their heart.

Q. How too can we the poetic perspective gain?
A. The poetry flows when we release the pain. From judgment our pain comes to be; when the moment's perfection we cannot see. Each moment in fullness, everything contains. There is nothing lacking, thus there is nothing to gain.

Q. When food is consumed, life is lost. Where is the poetry, when there is such a cost?
A. Many the illusions about the food that you eat; the belief of nutrition being an insurmountable need. A sacred ritual is how it should be seen: a communion with self through another being.

Q. How then, Master, can it be, that from the need to eat I can be free?
A. Food is only needed when there are unsung songs of the heart. It is not nourishment, but inspiration it imparts. When in surrender to existence's flow, the freedom from the need to eat you shall know.

Q. When our lives in surrender are fully lived, what benefits then shall eating give?
A. As all else you experience, it awakens within, the inspiration for the next notes you must sing. Eat then in silence that you may hear, the

feelings food evokes, that your steps may be clear. A guidance it is for the inspired life, softly it whispers, light as a sigh.

Q. What shall I do Master, if I cannot hear?
A. Though the mind may not know, to the body it shall be clear.

The Dream within the Dream

Q. Tell us now Master, of the worlds of the dream. The place where we go at night when we sleep…much time we spend there, yet unreal they seem.

A. Awake or asleep, both are a dream. For in your endless existence, they are images on a screen.

Q. Of what does the screen exist and how can we be free?

A. Of imagined building blocks, which consist of light and frequency. Tools are they, not the prison they seem. Tyrants they became because you believed the dream.

Q. What is the difference between our sleep and state of awakening?

A. The sleep in which you travel, like pilgrims in the night, is the soul's homecoming. The awake state of the day is the body's domain.

Q. And what of the spirit, where does it reign; in the time of our dreaming or the wakefulness of the day?

A. When sleep is so deep, that no dreams do you keep; no images remain when you awake, then you journeyed into spirit's states.

Q. How do we release the ties that bind, the belief in their realness held in our mind?

A. In the day, upon the stage you play. Know it is unreal, but act your part. It is for enjoyment; let lightness fill your heart. As you close your eyes when nighttime falls, journey not into the mirrors, the dream worlds that call. Dissolve the character and masks you hide behind. Return to the timelessness in which you reside.

Q. How then Master, shall this be done?

A. With intent and by remembering you are One. Like a current in the ocean of shoreless seas, without ending or beginning have you ever been.

Q. What is holy and what is profane? What shall we worship and what shall we disdain?
A. Holy or profane, but the flickering of light and shadow on the imagined fabric of time are they.

Q. Is it not wise to shun the murderer and revere the sage?
A. Shun the notes of life that are not yours to sing. Seek the inspiration that the sage may bring. But know that both have equal worth, for one brings order and from the other chaos is birthed. Chaos, when from an eternal perspective seen, is but the destructuring of what has been.

Q. But why must destructuring occur without grace? Why, in the beauty of life, must violence take place?
A. The forceful change violently wrought, breaks stagnant patterns of beliefs that are taught. In fluid surrender and a trusting heart, wherever you go, shall violence depart.

Q. When there is no aspect of life we should give more value to, when asked to choose, what shall we do?
A. The choice that is yours to make will inevitable seem, if your mind is clear and your heart free of needs.

Q. What can ease the burden of man?
A. A change in perspective and attitude can. The burdens he carries are made through time. Live fully in the moment; leave the past behind. See through the eyes of your eternal being, and the bumps on the road will be less than they seemed.

Q. Should we withdraw from the complexity of the crowds and the man-made societies?
A. Whenever you live in duality, and you think one pole more valuable than the other can be, you bring opposition by strengthening polarity. Depth of living comes from complexity. Its challenges bring vitality. Stagnation could come from simplicity.

Q. When both are valued equally, how should we combine them in harmony?
A. Cease to strive, outcomes to achieve, that awareness may grow of the details you see. To the complexity of the day, they bring the beauty of simplicity.

Q. Tell us now Master of cosmic life, if you can. What the cosmos is, we wish to understand.
A. The cosmos, like a disc around you lies, is a labyrinth in disguise. Not much more than lines in the sand. In four quadrants it lies, though unknown by man.

Q. How is it divided into four quadrants?
A. By walls of guilt and pain of the past. The body, soul and two levels of spirit are they. None of them are real – just acts in a play. Serious they seem in guiding your way. Through pain they prod you to walk the maze.

Q. How can we be free of such a painful play? How can we walk another way?
A. Stuck in the process, life has seemed. But more than a game it has never been. The soul, body and spirit are veils that enshroud infinity; to encapsulate a moment of eternity. Like a bucket in the ocean holds a fraction of the endless sea, so has duality framed unspeakable poetry.

Q. What purpose has been served by this illusional trinity?

A. It has tried to capture the grandeur of life's pageantry. The way the bucket thinks it can understand the endless sea and shifting sands. Each has a different perspective to see life unfold. Spirit is the one that the whole maze beholds. Physical life can only white light see. Soul's perspective, the black light between the lines has been.

Q. Why has there been great catastrophes that dwell like ghosts in the minds of humanity?

A. Like a dotted line that does not smoothly flow, man can only the white light and a broken line know. Of beginnings and endings does it consist. When vision changes, graceful change will exist.

Q. How can we increase our ability, the unfolding perfection of life to see?

A. Perception allows graceful change, but when we give meaning to what is seen, then it is maintained. Judgments keep the old in place. Thinking we know, prevents changing with grace. Power comes from letting go; power is lost when we think we know.

Q. What are these mirrors, of which the matrices are comprised, but a multi-perspective observing the eye?

A. For this they were intended, but forgotten their purpose became. Instead, as we believed them to be real, they began a tyrannical reign. Only by their combined perspectives, can clarity be gained. From their separate functioning, linear time came.

Q. What is the purpose of the multitudes of life?

A. You cannot see directly a beam of light. But when dust particles are there, the beams are visible to your sight. To the Infinite, aspects of Itself are seen in the multitude of living beings. The matrices are a window through which the light streams. Your body, soul and spirit are a frame for your eternal being.

Q. Having this knowledge, how must we each other see?
A. You are the particles of dust and the light of the beam; the roots and the trunk and the leaves of the tree. The leaves still live even as they fly free. The One Being sustains them, as It does the tree.

Q. What use is language, the words that we speak?
A. Like the particles of dust, the Infinite speaks in between. In their gaps is the unspeakable revealed. Hear not with your ears. See not with your eyes. For what can they reveal but imagined lies? It is behind the appearances that eternal truth lies.

Q. Master, I cannot comprehend. Of my body, soul and spirit, is this the end?
A. More dust particles are they that reveal the Infinite's face. In the game of self-observation, they have their place. When programs bind them they cannot show the Infinite's presence you wish to know. They are like a finger that points at the moon's luminosity: it is not the finger but the moon you must see.

Q. But they bring discouragement and pain?
A. Only if you in the illusion of the tyranny remain. Know the truth of your eternal being; like the ray of light, immovable it seems. Only within its presence, can the dust particles be. At no time can the window of the matrices have tyranny. All reality will change when from this illusion you are free.

Gods, Angels and Demons –
The Seer's Wisdom

Q. Master, tell us of the angels we revere, and of demons, which we fear.

A. Ask not of that which you yourselves have made, though of demons you are afraid and to angels you have prayed. Through your judgments of good and bad did they arise. That one pole can have more value than another is one of illusion's greatest lies.

Q. Of what then Master are angels comprised?

A. They hold the light; all that can be grasped by mind. They are holders of order and order is wisdom of days gone by.

Q. And demons then, what function have they?

A. The embodiment of chaos are they. Order is that which wishes to maintain grids of knowledge of bygone days. Man values order's predictability. Chaos is suppressed by humanity. From having only order, there would be a structured society. This brings stagnation and evokes calamities.

Q. But order brings peace and chaos pain. How can we from chaos, benefits gain?

A. Demons hold chaos, which otherwise would have to manifest in human lives. A purpose they serve until man can see, that chaos is nothing more than destructuring. Life is like a flow, like the seething seas, not a static construction that is the same eternally. The answer to avoiding catastrophes lies not in clinging to order, but through balance within.

Q. Will this the existence of demons negate?
A. Yes, but then you must also the angels forsake. They represent the rejected parts of yourself: your self-made heaven and inner hell. Look beyond the judgments taught by humanity, and see with the eyes of eternity. The thunder and the sunshine, all are part of the poetry.

Q. As we proclaim the worth of angels, what then? Do demons then too walk among men?
A. One cannot add weight to one side of a scale without causing imbalance that the cosmos would feel. In nature too, imbalance you will see.

Q. How would this be?
A. Predators would in numbers decrease. Grass-eaters would multiply and barren lands would increase.

Q. Surely you do not mean that we should demons embrace?
A. No, for in the world of men they have no place. Each serves a purpose that benefits all life. But each to their own realms must be confined.

Q. When will such separation ever cease?
A. When linear time shall no longer be, then shall all creatures be redeemed.

Q. What of the gods, do they exist in realms on high?
A. Among humanity they hide. Forgotten have they that they are of a more evolved race. The contracted vision of humankind has erased their origins from their minds. Different is their DNA. Their great capacities hide away. But they have come to ease men's plight by restoring to humanity greater sight.

Q. Whence did they come to dwell among men?

A. The question should not be from where, but from when. The Earth has always been their home. Through time they've come, together or alone.

Q. What is the advantage of gods who have lost their memories?
A. The wayshowers are they of humanity. Through the overcomings of their lives they bring liberty.

Q. Why have we not of this been told?
A. Why remember dreams of old? In living from realness, you discard all roles. Personalities form from the stories of ages gone by. They become your prison cell in time. Experience instead the world like a child; forget your ego and release your pride.

Q. When we accept all that on the stage of life plays, will angels and demons go away?
A. No, they will simply another role play.

Q. If aspects within us these beings have made, whose aspects are we within life's play?
A. Life within the matrix is linearly made; when you end its illusion, all this goes away. Within the matrix, from the gods you came, and other kingdoms from humanity's reflections came. When you are free from duality, it will no more be the same.

Q. How will it be when we are free? Will linear becoming no longer reign?
A. Each creature exists eternally. For another to create it, there is no need. When the blindness of the matrix is gone, it will be seen.

Q. But then again, many are they?

A. No, just the One Life at play. Of the cells in your body are you comprised. Thus many you are, though it seems as one to the eyes. With the Infinite it is not the same, since there is no such thing as space, but it is an image with which to explain how all can seem separate, then one again.

When forms and roles are kept in our memories, beings cannot evolve fluidly. We keep them in place with old memories. Like flickers of light and shade across eternity, they dance to the Song of Eternity.

Q. Tell us oh Master, of that which we see; how our environment a mirror has come to be?
A. The senses of man as perspectives were made, instead tyrants they became. Their preferences of how they wished life to be, prevented their ability of eternal expression to see. The observer and the observed became one, the existence of the environment as a mirror had begun.

Q. Master, how can we from such illusion be free? How can we the Eternal and Infinite see?
A. In between the sensory input you shall find the Infinite's face. In the silence between the words, Infinite communication takes place. Let me explain what words cannot provide; that which as truth must be felt inside. The Infinite and finite are both the same; one cannot more value than the other retain. All that exists is Infinite Life; within Its presence nothing else abides. The illusion of the finite, which in our life we find, is part of the aspects of self we reject inside.

Q. Yet shallow are the lives of those who choose to live only in the finite. Thus how must we see it, what must we do?
A. To transcend this duality, your judgment you must lose. Do not place value only on eternity, neglecting the moment's wondrous beauty. What is eternity, but a moment without boundary?

Q. Time is movement, this you have taught, but deeper understanding of its motion we have sought.

A. It is part of the Infinite's dance of joy and passion. It circles like wheels, and like an arrow it flies in its expression. On the disc of life, like currents within the infinite sea, it moves in different ways throughout eternity.

Q. A subjective experience within the vastness of our being, how can time be measured or space be seen?

A. In the contradiction of life, measurements are the tool of an arrogant fool. When the wise look beyond the game, no measurement of time and space remains. Space is defined by the measurement of time which flickers and plays upon the eternal stage.

Q. I feel, oh Master, in deep despair. Within me both light and darkness are there. How can I conquer the objectionable within? How can a life of poise and mastery begin?

A. The life you seek will be begun, when both aspects of yourself are accepted as one. Your anger fights for its place in the sun. That which is suppressed, stronger becomes.

Q. How shall I prevent its damage in my life?

A. Fly like the eagle high in the sky. Observe how you express the anger when it does arise. Mastery does not suppress emotions' flow, but directs the way in which the expression should go.

Q. What of despair, Master, why is it there?

A. It arises when you forsake the truth of your being; when the adventure of life cannot be seen. Life withers when external validation you seek, it flourishes when an eternal perspective you keep. Society demands that your existence be justified, but no thread can be removed from the intricate pattern of life. Behind the mask with which you hide, the omniscience of the ages eternally abides. A sacred portal into Infinity, this you are throughout eternity.

Q. Why is it Master, wherever I go, that a deep grief within travels with me also? A sad note lingers in the most joyous refrain, in moments of rejoicing yet there is pain?
A. I tell you now whence this comes, pain is the result of forgetting we are one. The pain of separation, from self-alienation is born. As you journey, it lingers like an unwanted thorn.

Q. From what have we separated that this would be so? How can contentment replace the pain that we know?
A. Man has imagined that he could be separated from the natural world's harmony. Imbalance within nature and within humanity is the result of this rift that has come to be. Man finds hostility in nature, but this is caused by his separative beliefs.

Q. Was it always thus, Master please tell, or did man in harmony with nature once dwell?
A. Many times among humanity, forgetfulness came and with it, global calamities. At one with nature, hardiness grows. In reconnection, healthful resilience is known. A neutral energy through the natural man flows. As a grounding rod, the gift of fertility he bestows. A blessing to the land he becomes, when he has reunited with nature as one.

Q. How can we too these blessings know as our connection with nature is once again known?
A. Cease to wear footwear that insulates. Let it be made from material that with the Earth resonates.

Q. Like leather or wood? Would they be good?

A. Yes, but walk barefoot upon the land whenever you can. Let your children in nature, spend much time, that eyesight through depth-perception may improve, as they run and climb.

In communion with nature, the archetypal spirits of nature can be known; of earth, fire and wind, as well as all waters that flow.

Q. Will they then our allies become? To call on for assistance, when more rain is needed or more sun?
A. This you can do, but there is a higher way: Relationship with allies still divides and separates. Once you've found the archetypes without, let them resonate within. When the outer and inner are one, a life of miracles begins. Know the song of the water through the flow in your veins. As you emphasize it through awareness, you will call the rains.

All aspects of nature within you have their counterparts. The pulsing sun at the center of the Earth, is the beating of your heart.

Q. What of the stones that around us lie?
A. Like the bones in your body, secrets they hide.

Q. And the plants, can we know them too?
A. In telepathic communication they speak to you. As a thought within your thoughts, their voice you'll hear. Be still and receptive and it shall become clear.

Q. Of what can plants teach, what will they say?
A. They tell of feelings – masters of pure emotions are they.

Q. What of gemstones and stones – what do they know?
A. History and knowledge do they hold. Stones keep the stories of long ago. Gemstones hold aware moments, most dear, of encountering the real when eternity became clear. Stones hold the light of linear time.

Gemstones are windows through which a glimpse of the Infinite you will find.

Q. You have taught us Master that through diamonds we can wield the most potent alchemy…
A. Yes, but the alchemy of plant fragrances has more potency.

Q. Why can animals thrive without needing tools in their natural state, but man is dependent on the implements he creates?
A. Animals to specific regions are confined. The tools of man bring freedom to humankind. With them he can travel in the deepest snow, yet the jungles and the deserts too he can know.

Tools should be seen with gratitude in this light. Instead, an arrogance they have brought to humankind. Through his lenses he can see with the eagle's eye. Like the falcon, in his machines, he soars through the sky, and like the whale beneath the ocean, he dives.

Honor the gifts the animals know, as through your ingenuity you make them your own. Do not separate from nature through a sense of superiority, but appreciate their diverse contribution through increased sensitivity.

You are their steward to tend and protect. Treat well the garden of your Earthly home with love and respect.

Relationships

Q. Tell us now Master, of the relationships of man; how to bring them into oneness, if we can.

A. First you must know where they began. The origin of relationship is the spirit, body and soul – before they began, just oneness did you know. Before they formed, like a candle in the sun, you knew that with Source you were one.

Q. How should we to these relate?

A. Know their controlling games, but live from your core. Behind the appearances, know there's so much more.

Q. But why do you then teach us how to work with daily life, when we should ignore it and gain deeper sight?

A. Imagine a table, with clutter filled. But under the mess, lies a priceless pearl. Create first order, that you may see the priceless pearl that you seek.

Q. In relationship, what then is real? The alchemy we create or the love that we feel?

A. When deep and with pure intent, then real it is for sure. But often the real, by games is obscured. Identify the areas where control yet can be found, where a desire for specific outcomes yet abounds. Then know such realities are not for you, to allow yourself to indulge them, you must refuse.

Seek in each other the gifts you bring. Let inspiration you gain, cause your heart to sing. Through keen awareness, anew you must see, each other's true essence of majesty.

Q. Must every encounter yield these discoveries or just those who are close to me?

A. In every person it is yourself that you see. Your loved ones yield more clarity. In your shared sexuality, your partner lets you see eternity.

Communication and Relationship

Q. Why does such strife between people exist? What must we accept and what must we resist?

A. Suffering, when shared, is but an emphasis of the common bond of man that like a field exists. Experiences that are jointly shared are a meeting point of the unique perspectives that are there.

Q. And how then must communication be seen?

A. Communication between two individual beings, each in an entirely different reality, seems at times like an impossibility. The gift a shared experience imparts, is that it invokes the common resonance of the heart.

Q. Thus the feelings behind our words make them come alive. Communication must be felt rather than contrived?

A. When hearing and speaking both become an extension of ourselves, we communicate as one.

Q. Is there aught that we must get clear on how to speak and how to hear?

A. In a silenced mind, another's words can be received. Breathing is important when you speak. Like one who sings, your speech should go. On the outbreath only, let them flow. For words with power to come forth, from the full pranic tube they must be drawn.

Q. The pranic tube that from the base of the spine does go?

A. That is only the part commonly known. Prana from within the ground does flow; the tube begins a hand length below. From under the ground, in a straight line to the spine, the unknown part of the tube you'll find.

Q. From a hand length below the ground to the base of the spine, why has this part of the pranic tube been unknown to humankind?

A. It is what you use when claimed by death, or when asleep upon your bed. The full use of the pranic tube can be reclaimed by breath.

Q. Tell us Master, how should we receive the knowledge that another speaks?

A. Knowledge is of accumulated facts comprised. Gathered over years, it is highly prized. Man has been addicted to complexity, thus values more that which is obtained with difficulty. That which is in an instant to awareness shown, knowledge cannot with much learning know.

Q. Why then Master, is this so?

A. Knowledge is purely electric and can only see a contracted perspective of reality. Awareness has an emotional component too, and can reveal a broader perspective to you.

Q. How can we the truth of another's words discern? How can we the difference between the real and the unreal learn?

A. Real and unreal is not what it seems. It is simply a matter of where your attention has been. Within the limitlessness of your eternal being, whatever is focused on becomes real. That which lies outside the scope of what you see, becomes classified as the unreal.

Q. Realness therefore cannot be, when a subjective standard is all it seems. Does focus then determine reality?

A. Through contracted focus, awareness is decreased; by emphasis through resonance of the heart, awareness is increased. Create your reality through the heart and higher consciousness it will impart.

Q. What hardship from the focus of the mind can come?

A. Its contracted focus excludes, and the excluded parts of life become our opposition.

Strong Suits and Faults

Q. If a fault is our enemy within, an unexpressed part that opposition brings, then how must the resolution of this begin?

A. Our strong suits are valued, they hide our faults, their emphasis takes energy away from the unexpressed parts. From our emphasized strong suits, identities arise. Effortless renewal of experience is denied. Trapped by our strong suits, we're cut off from resources' limitless supply.

Q. Our mistakes then must be valued too?

A. Yes, begin by understanding why they're found within you.

Q. Should we value and focus on our strong suits of past times gone by?

A. To do so is to define yourself by the conduct of past times. A strong suit is merely that which you emphasize. What we suppress and reject as faults is categorized.

Q. But faults are not suppressed when they're in front of our eyes.

A. A substitute expression; that which is fake, replaces the unexpressed to be lived in its place. Of a belief program does it consist. Where belief systems are, dysfunction exists.

Q. How can we see the value in the faults we hold, when they're upside down to our being, which makes them hostile, we are told?

A. Without either the judgment of heart or of mind, nothing is either hostile or benign. An up or down side from our judgment is formed. That which is hostile, from our rejection is born. Faults and weaknesses are just part of our eternal journey, steered by the resonance of the heart.

Q. What other judgments from our hearts are formed; what flawed perception from our mind is born?

A. We overvalue oneness because of the peace it brings. We undervalue the separation of duality, because it challenges us through its complexity.

Q. What can be done to find peace of heart and peace of mind?

A. Peace is disrupted by imbalance within. It is judgment that always imbalance brings.

Q. Besides ensuring that judgment is released, what else can we do to live in peace?

A. To breathe[1] from the pranic tube's full extent, creates neutrality that can catastrophes prevent.

Like a lightning rod that grounds electricity, for yourself and your environment, you avert calamities.

Q. Of what use are faults; of what benefit are they?

A. The adversity they create, indicate what directions you need to change along the way. But not just teachers of adversity are they, but instruments of manifestation and creativity.

Q. What we don't express today, may yet tomorrow be so. Is a fault then only a strong suit we don't yet know?

A. When fully expressed, yes, it is so.

Q. Then how do we know what way to go?

A. The adventure in your heart will lead you and the poetry of your soul. When you live the spirit of adventure and wonderment, and the perspectives of eternity as well as poetry, you become part of an

1 See Book I, page 5, *The Seven Sacred Breaths of Eternal Life – The Arasatma Breathing Techniques.*

equation of alchemy. Then opened the gates of the magical worlds shall be.

Q. When we once again the magical kingdoms see, what shall the effect on them then be? Shall we know more peace?
A. Appreciative awareness is a quality that helps them thrive, when bestowed by humanity. The more your love for them grows, the more vitality they shall know. Peace is not in external conditions found, but in embracing the unpredictable does it abound.

Q. How do we communicate with our own inner being, when the multi-levels of existence different songs sing?
A. Through love, trust, gratitude and praise shall an empathic connection be maintained.

Q. What causes this communication to be blocked?
A. Through the guilt you feel, these avenues are locked. Trust that all is as it should be, and from the guilt over the past shall you be free.

Q. In remembering our choices, how can we see how the things that we did, were meant to be?
A. In a cosmos where there is no right or wrong, how can there be 'wrong' choices then within the One Being?

Q. But Master, what of suffering; how does it fit in the eternal scheme?
A. Suffering is no longer so when we no longer resist. Then its true nature as a pressure to guide us, alone exists. Choices that now seem wrong, awakened deeper expression within. A prerequisite for a new level of awareness to begin.

Sa-huna Satma

The Breaths of Higher Consciousness

Ki arasha nenuch va-u ste-ara,
nunit sa-huna ba-ur anasavi.

When freedom from the wheel of life is
attained, the birth of a higher consciousness
is likewise.

The Breathing Techniques of Sa-huna Satma

When doing the Sa-huna Satma Breaths you will need:

- A yoga mat, pillow or chair so you can sit comfortably for the duration of the 144 breaths.
- The following 4 Wheels of Higher Consciousness:
  - *The Wheel of Perpetual Regeneration through Trust in Self-sovereignty*
  - *The Atlantean Wheel of Angels*
  - *The Lemurian Wheel of Angels*
  - *The Wheel of Combined Realities*
- Place these wheels in a stack, beneath where you are sitting (they may be laminated to preserve them). Wheel 1 is on top, Wheel 4 is at the bottom.
- On top of the stack of 4 wheels, place the *Equation to Combine the Frequency-based DNA Strand with the Light-based DNA Strand.*
- On top of that equation, place: *The Equation for the Ceremony of Incorruptibility.*
- The music created for the breathing techniques.
- The *144 Tones of Purity,* along with the sigils and angel names.

Note: Prior to doing the Sa-huna Satma Breaths, it is important that you have completed all 3 Levels of the Arasatma Breaths and the Nevi-Satma, Twelve Breaths of Proxy. The Nevi-Satma Breaths should have been practised at least once, followed by a day's break, before doing the Sa-huna Satma Breaths.

To reduce the effects of detoxification on the body following these breath exercises, it is advisable that you have a day of rest and drink plenty of water.

Posture:
- During these breaths, you may either sit on the floor or on a chair with the stack of wheels and the alchemical equations below you. You will remain seated for all 144 breaths.
- Throughout the entire exercise it is important that your spine is straight.
- Your legs may be crossed if you are sitting on the floor or flat on the floor with your feet together if you are sitting on a chair.
- Your hands may be placed however is most comfortable.

The Tones of Purity:
- As you do the breaths, you will be reading the names of the Tones of Purity (one tone for each breath) and focusing on the relevant sigil.
- Call the name of the angel associated with each tone.
- When doing the breathing exercises by yourself, it is easy to lose your place as you move through all 144. Placing the pages with the Sigils and Tones of Purity in front of you and moving your finger down them one by one as you read them, is advised.
- In group sessions, the leader can call out the Tones of Purity but it is still important that each participant can look at the relevant sigil.

The Breaths:
- There are 144 in-breaths (to a count of 3) and 144 out-breaths (to a count of 3). The gaps between the in- and out-breaths are small. Make sure you do not hyperventilate. If you get dizzy, lie down and take a break. The wheels and sigils act as a power source.
- With each breath, move your finger to the relevant sigil and read (or have someone else read) the corresponding Tone of Purity. The

Tone of Purity should be read on the in-breath and you can look at the sigil during the out-breath. Moving the eyes from left to right is beneficial in helping to clear the impurities of the past. (A Powerpoint presentation of the Tones and sigils could also be used and will have the same effect).

- On the last (144th) out-breath, force the breath out in a long deep exhalation, emptying your lungs completely. When it seems as though no air is left in the lungs, force out another short puff of air.

The Wheels of the Sa-huna Satma Breaths

Chaba huchna sa-una savit, Ma-at na-unestra cha-una ba urasat vinesbi.

Wheels within wheels they turn, bringing freedom from the wheel of time.

From the Scroll of Manusat

The Wheel of Perpetual Regeneration
through Trust in Self-Sovereignty

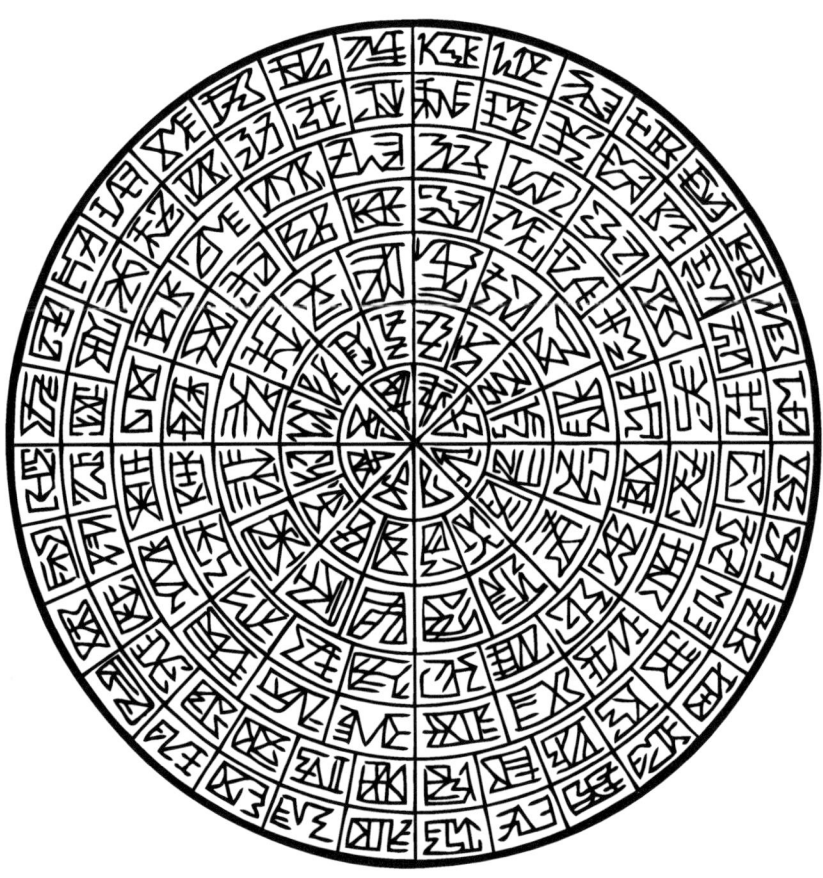

Understanding the Sigils of the Wheel

The 144 sigils of which the wheel is comprised, embody the 144 tones of purity found in higher cosmic life. Each frequency or tone is represented by an angelic order. The term 'higher' as used when referring to consciousness or angelic orders does not refer to higher frequency, which makes reality less dense and more etheric. It refers to more highly evolved complexity and refinement of expression.

Purity refers to the unobstructed expression of Infinite Intent as expressed through finite individuations.

The Meaning of the Wheel

The impurities of life, born of resistance created by the value judgments of belief systems, separate an individuation from Source. The removal of these obstructions through the restoration of the tones of purity, re-establishes the limitless supply of resources of our eternal existence.

The result of dwelling within the eternal supply of resources, is the return to our natural state of timeless and perpetual regeneration. To achieve this, we must relinquish the belief that we must be externally supplied and nourished. We must trust that, as an aspect of eternal and Infinite Life, we are able to supply ourselves in absolute self-sovereignty.

The Placement of the Wheel

The wheel is placed on top of the stack of four wheels, which means that as the first wheel, its effects will be felt first.

The goal of the Sa-huna Satma Breaths is to create the integration of body and soul, overcoming the cycles of life and death and functioning as a resurrected being. This allows perpetual regeneration to take place.

The first step in this process entails the purified expression of body and soul – the function of this wheel.

The Wheel of the Atlantean Angels
(also known as the Wheel of the Divine Masculine)

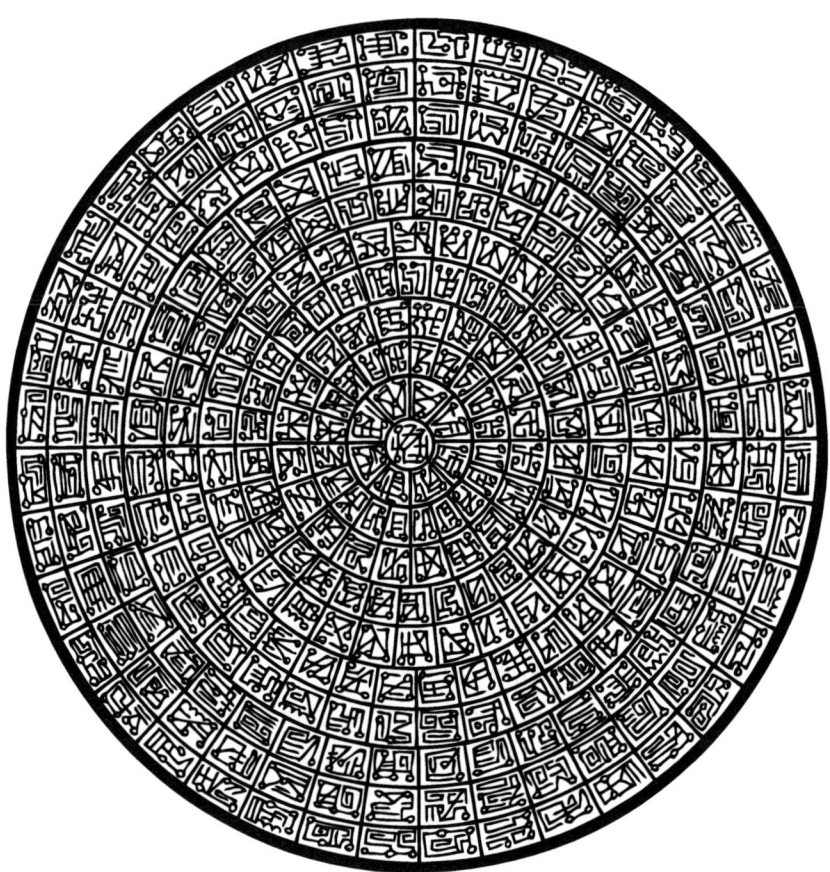

Understanding the Sigils of the Wheel

In an advanced being, living from an evolved level of consciousness, the two strands of DNA actually consist of clusters of 300 strands each. One strand is more electric and the other more magnetic.

The 300 electric strands are representative of the 300 perception-based principles of the divine masculine, present within each being. The Wheel of the Atlantean Angels is comprised of 300 sigils representing the full expression of the divine masculine (see Appendix I for the difference between sigils and symbols).

The Meaning of the Wheel

The Atlantean Angels are a specific group of 300 angelic orders embodying the 300 insights of the masculine principles. Insights are information-based and therefore electric in nature. These were specifically studied by the Atlantean civilization, especially since they were determining factors in the nature of light as the cosmos moved through 300 positions in its massive orbit.

The Placement of the Wheel

This wheel, placed second from the top, is the second influence that will be felt during the Sa-huna Satma breathing techniques. Having been purified by the top wheel, the electric-based DNA strand is now challenged and stimulated into full expression of all 300 aspects.

The Wheel of the Lemurian Angels
(also known as the Wheel of the Divine Feminine)

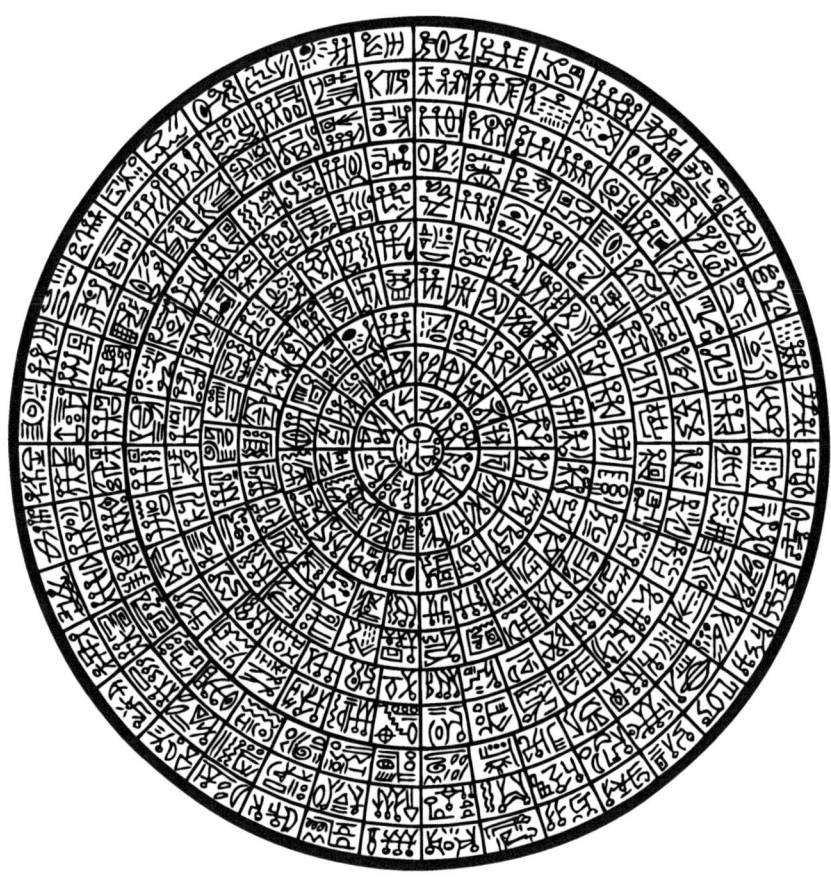

The Meaning of the Sigils of the Wheel

As Atlantis represented the masculine archetype of the Earth, so Lemuria (also called the Mother Land) represented the feminine archetype. The sigils on the Wheel represent the 300 archetypal aspects or frequency-based traits of the divine feminine.

The magnetic, feminine strand of DNA in an advanced being is a cluster of 300 strands representing the 300 principles of the divine feminine. The purpose of this wheel is to stimulate the activation of their expression.

The Meaning of the Wheel

Physical life is more light-based and electrical. Soul is magnetic and frequency-based. The soul components, represented by this wheel, must be expressed in an integrated way within physical life, else soul becomes an externalized aggressor towards the body, and the tug of war between life and death rages. The soul frequencies' expression in life is restored by this wheel.

The Placement of the Wheel

The soul frequencies, like all magnetic components, hold memories – the ghosts of the past. The top wheel purifies the memories of this wheel, as well as emotional injuries of the previously suppressed feminine expression within us. The balancing, healing and expressing of the purified masculine and feminine is needed before combining both inner aspects into a resurrected being.

The Wheel of Combined Realities

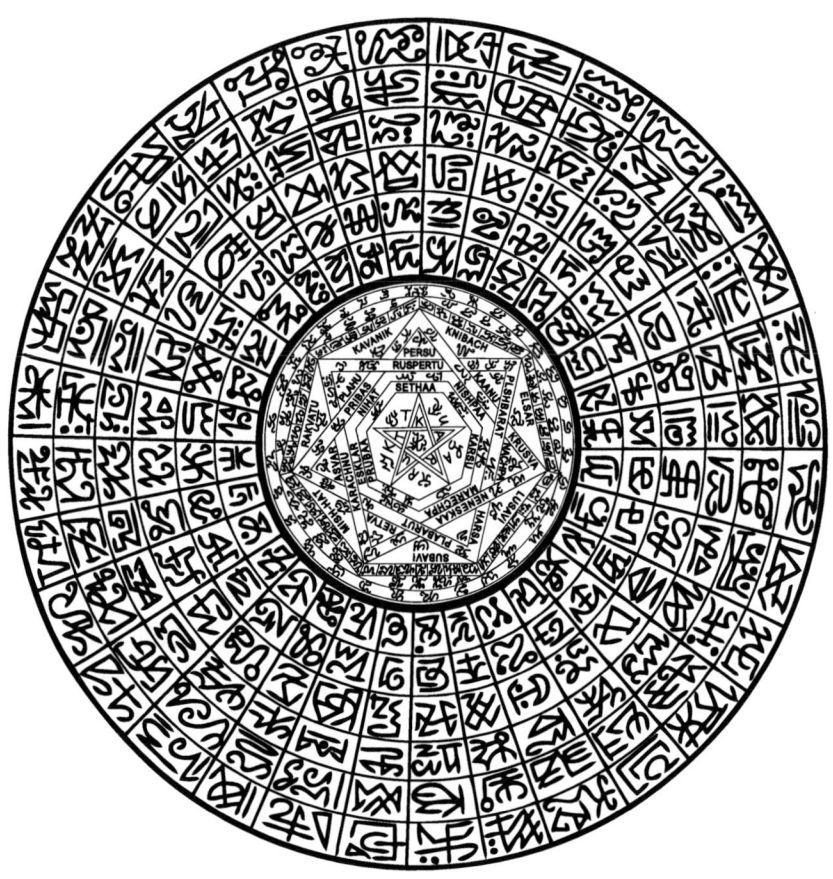

The Meaning of the Sigils on the Wheel

This powerful wheel consists of rings of sigils of physical alchemy around the center sigil, called the Sigil of Blahut. The Sigil of Blahut represents the soul, and the physical alchemical sigils represent the body.

The Sigil of Blahut

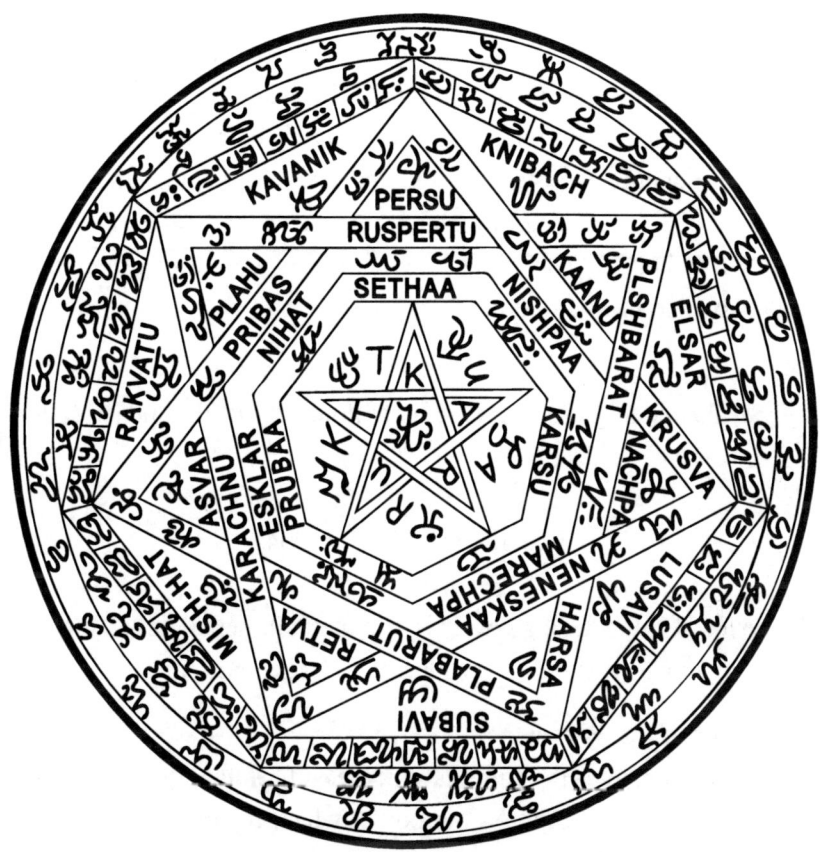

Excerpt from the *Lemurian Records of the 300 Angels of Frequency*
The Sigil of Ameth, used by ancient alchemists, has kept the angels of the black light (refined and unseen light) in a state of lower consciousness. The Sigil of Blahut sets the angelic realms free to live from their higher consciousness. To do this, the old angels are replaced with those of higher consciousness. The Lemurian records have preserved the names of the 300 higher angels to be given at the end of time as we know

it. They usher in a new form of time – the eternal moment. Their 300 insights are reminders of what needs to be known to make this transition on Earth.

The Meaning of the Wheel

Physical alchemy can leverage the equation of two parts added together up to 96. One plus one can equal 96. The outer rings represent this alchemical transmutation that can take place in the body. When dealing with the alchemical potencies of frequency, one plus one can be leveraged to 300. The Sigil of Blahut represents this ability. By adding these two alchemical capacities together and by combining them into a single wheel, a new equation forms:

Physical Alchemy (96) + Alchemical Potencies of Frequency (300)

=

Resurrected Matter (1054)

The result of this wheel's power is exponential, beneficial change and becoming our own supply of resources for regeneration.

Placement of the Wheel

The Wheel represents the culmination; the end result of the combination of the other three wheels. As the power wheel for the Sa-huna Satma breaths, it is placed at the bottom of the stack.

The Equation of Resurrected Matter

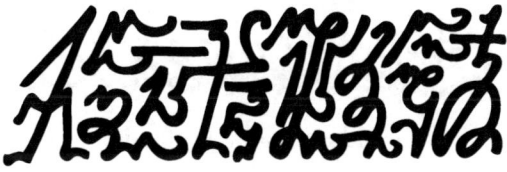

Physical Alchemy

+

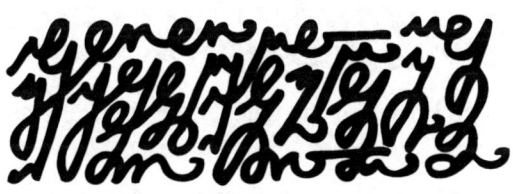

Alchemical Potencies of Frequency

=

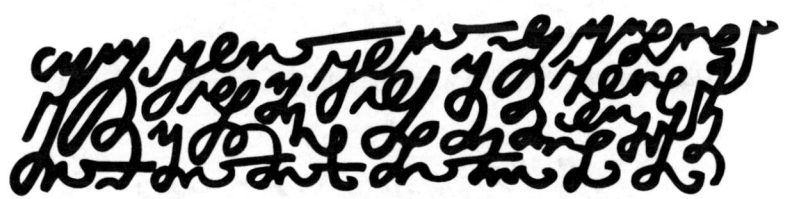

Resurrected Matter

The Equation to Combine the Frequency-based DNA Strand with the Light-based DNA Strand

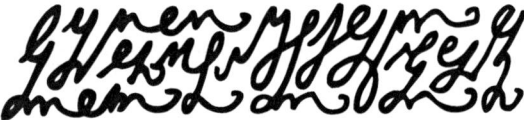

Remembering the Indescribable Perfection of the One Life

+

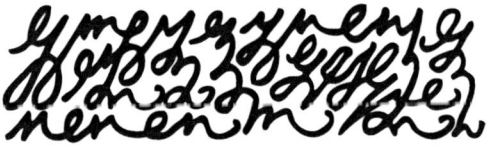

The Awakened Poetry of the One Life Expressing as the Many

+

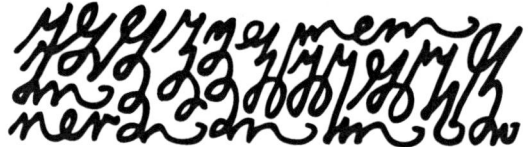

The Harmonious Interaction of the Many Expressing as the One

+

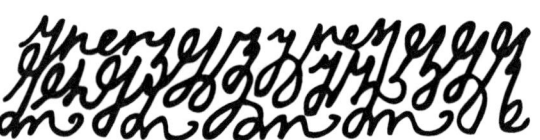

Remembered Indivisibility of Eternal Beingness

=

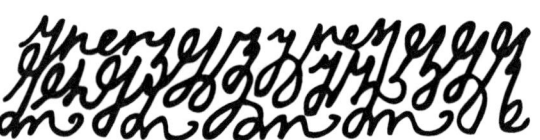

The Merging of the One and the Many for the Fruition and Release of the Spiritual Gifts of Evolved DNA

The Equation for the Ceremony of Incorruptibility

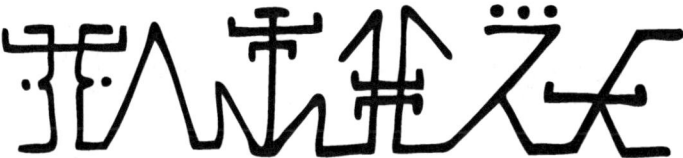

The Ushering in of a Reign of Purity through Holy Proclamations

+

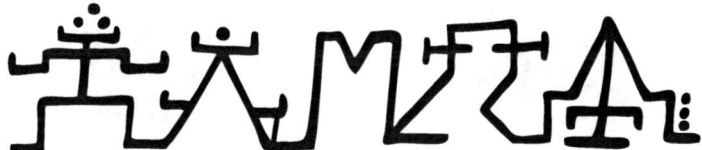

The Dissolving of Unholy Alliances of Existence

+

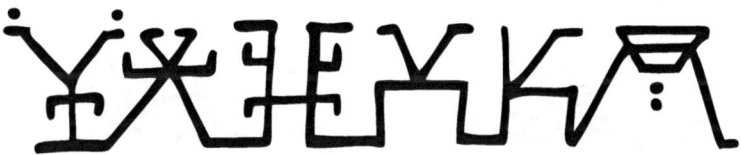

Illuminating the Fabric of Existence

=

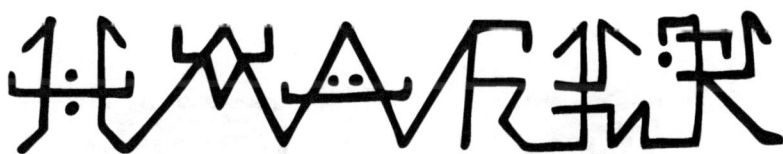

The Purification and Incorruptibility of Life

The 144 Tones of Purity

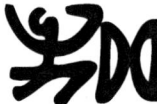

Angel – *Mesepe-iranat*

1. The original patterns of existence

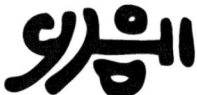

Angel – *Mesech-nunat*

5. Surrendered silent song

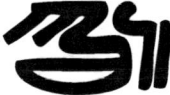

Angel – *Sihuch-raspahur*

2. Dynamic unfolding of purity

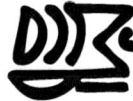

Angel – *Brivatu-eresvi*

6. Motionless movement

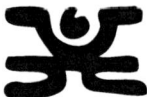

Angel – *Ninset-eklechve*

3. Removing illusion through perception

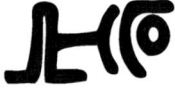

Angel – *Harstu-etrevi*

7. Limitless alchemy

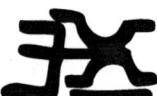

Angel – *Brurach-nivet*

4. Fluidly forming repatterning

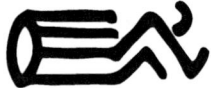

Angel – *Nasavi-hersetu*

8. Open-ended equations

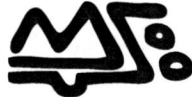

Angel – *Blivabich-beret*

9. Releasing the need for predictability

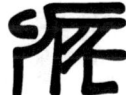

Angel – *Rasvabit-herstu*

10. Embracing patternless existence

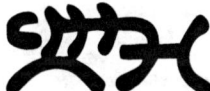

Angel – *Vravablik-misu*

11. Resolving illusory patterns of distortion

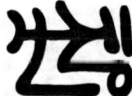

Angel – *Nanet-herseta*

12. Knowing truth to be the unfolding moment

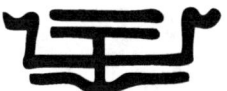

Angel – *Knanech-sitru*

13. Effortless expression of inevitability

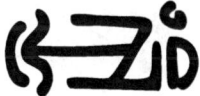

Angel – *Kravavit-velspa*

14. Moving beyond linear change

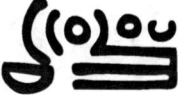

Angel – *Rukvabit-liset*

15. Releasing the need to know

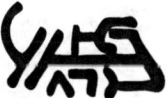

Angel – *Necvahur-akla*

16. Living from the eternal perspective

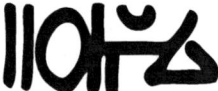

Angel – *Arus-harsava*

17. Releasing programmed
notions of purity

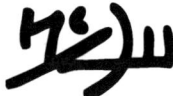

Angel – *Nestu-aklet*

18. Inspired opposites

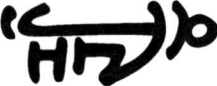

Angel – *Haravach-miset*

19. Releasing programs of
the physical

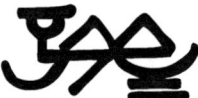

Angel – *Kliset-menetvi*

20. Releasing programs of the soul

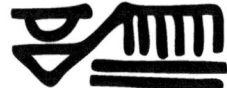

Angel – *Trebavich-setu*

21. Releasing programs of the
levels of spirit

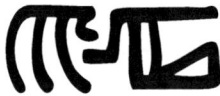

Angel – *Larasach-visabet*

22. Omniperspective immersal
into experience

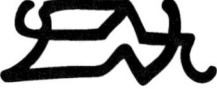

Angel – *Arta-minusech*

23. Releasing neediness through
dynamic balance

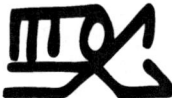

Angel – *Klahart-prasur*

24. Remembered oneness
within interaction

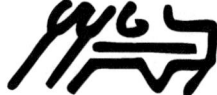

Angel – *Mishach-herestu*

25. Growing self-delight through adventure

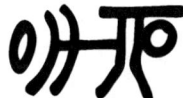

Angel – *Bribes-ruseter*

29. Creative dance of duality

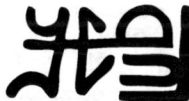

Angel – *Mespa-nespahur*

26. Releasing obsolete stories

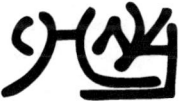

Angel – *Kersatu-plibahus*

30. Valued acceptance of light and shadow

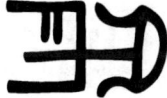

Angel – *Kersech-pritahur*

27. Knowing indivisibility

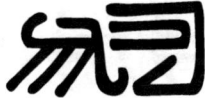

Angel – *Mesenech-sitrutve*

31. Fun-filled lightness of being

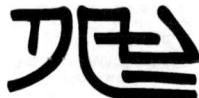

Angel – *Mespe-uhurasak*

28. Graceful immersal through non-resistance

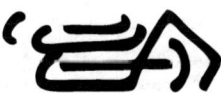

Angel – *Eskra-virabit*

32. Fractal change through Infinite expression

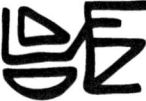

Angel – *Rutvi-sabahut*

33. Releasing the Cosmic Story

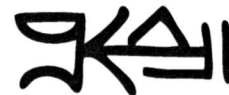

Angel – *Archtu-nenespavi*

37. Embracing change from the changeless self

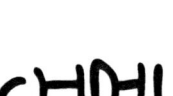

Angel – *Nensuk-arakrachve*

34. Releasing physical history

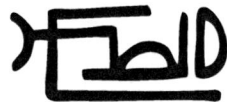

Angel – *Rutsat-plakplehur*

38. Transparent honesty

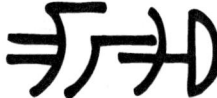

Angel – *Nesenukrava*

35. Omnipresent immediate expression

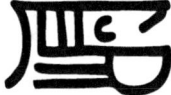

Angel – *Arska-eseklet-plahur*

39. Cooperation with the eternal dance

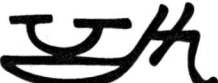

Angel – *Etre-barus-haresta*

36. Removing concepts of hierarchy through fusion

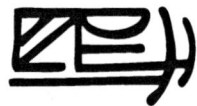

Angel – *Vilesblavat-skavi*

40. Uninterrupted unfoldment

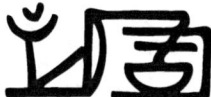

Angel – *Pereska-blihat-unas*

41. Compassionate interaction

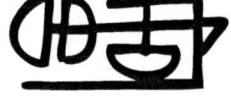

Angel – *Braruk-pilsh-bravi*

45. Releasing the dependency on verbal communication

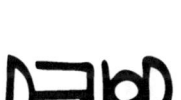

Angel – *Kriseta-una*

42. Agendaless co-habitation

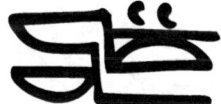

Angel – *Prihunat-sklaruch*

46. Openness to receive

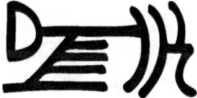

Angel – *Sihurat-anas*

43. Readiness for ingenious solutions

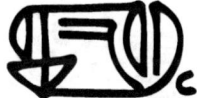

Angel – *Tri-unet-skelarut*

47. Uncompromising devotion to clarity

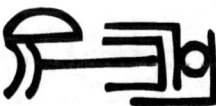

Angel – *Sparach-nusavet*

44. Childlike delight at the gift of existence

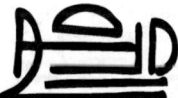

Angel – *Brisparvet-nusarek*

48. Formlessly forming the body anew always

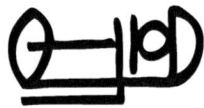

Angel – *Perenet-akla*

49. Thorough appreciation of omnipresent beauty

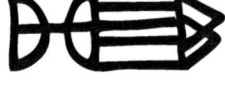

Angel – *Kiseret-suvata*

53. Releasing self-definitions

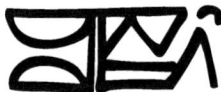

Angel – *Esebit-hunat*

50. Knowing the self as the many

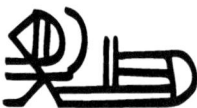

Angel – *Ersete-hunanach*

54. Wonderment through appreciation

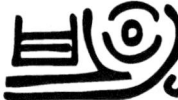

Angel – *Kesut-ararech*

51. Releasing the body as a reference point

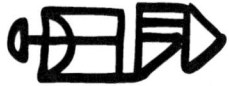

Angel – *Suhit-miseta*

55. Unencumbered journey

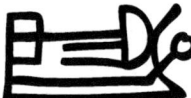

Angel – *Brisekla-pileshal*

52. Inclusive actions

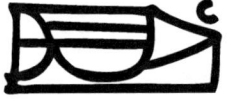

Angel – *Plavit-heresut*

56. Dissolving embedded programs

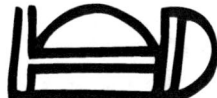

Angel – *Krinech-bluhet-aski*

57. Releasing protective
mechanisms

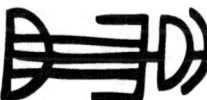

Angel – *Vibrat-hunanechvi*

58. Ruthless honesty with oneself

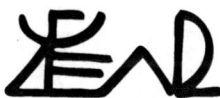

Angel – *Helsenut-plihar*

59. Knowing the concept of
possessions as a flow

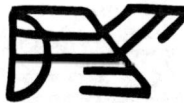

Angel – *Nanate-rukvahar*

60. Finding joy in the original
simplicity of self

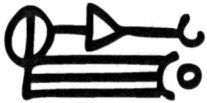

Angel – *Sursabich-mechnetu*

61. Passionate discoveries of
eternity in others

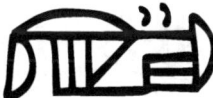

Angel – *Kuvanare-prehatur*

62. Flawless expression of
Infinite inevitability

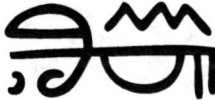

Angel – *Aruk-neseta*

63. Contributing creative artistry

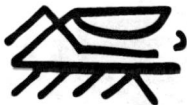

Angel – *Kavech-urat*

64. Purity through the poetic
perspective

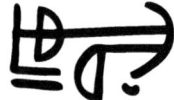

Angel – *Brihar-enesu*

65. Acknowledging knowing nothing

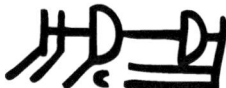

Angel – *Skavit-usbekla*

66. Seeing all existence as unknowable

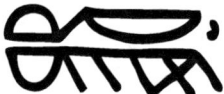

Angel – *Kelsuta-avanes*

67. Reverential journey

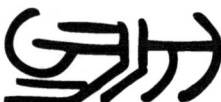

Angel – *Mirechsta-bruhatar*

68. Releasing shelters through trust

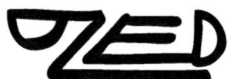

Angel – *Sihunet-akvabar*

69. Accepting existence as having neither guilt nor innocence

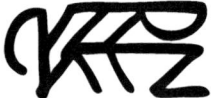

Angel – *Ekvehut-manasu*

70. Releasing the need to steer today by yesterday's wisdom

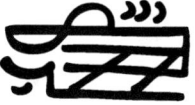

Angel – *Ritarat-nenusa*

71. Resting in activity

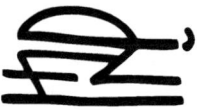

Angel – *Rukperevet-hivanech*

72. Purified dream states

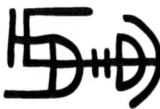

Angel – *Ruplekplahur-mishenut*

73. Purified awake states

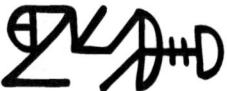

Angel – *Visetret-krananus*

77. Resonant harmony of the Infinite Being

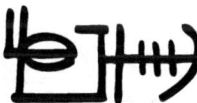

Angel – *Risberetuk-plivanu*

74. Valued contribution of the many to the one

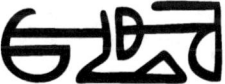

Angel – *Esebit-asklaha*

78. Refined nuances of enjoyment

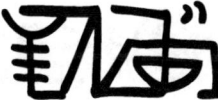

Angel – *Riseblechplavi*

75. Ageless expression

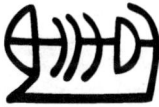

Angel – *Ukranenuk-sitrahur*

79. Undefinable knowingness

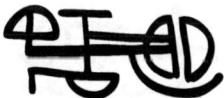

Angel – *Nunaresplaha*

76. Fusion of opposites

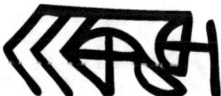

Angel – *Kasuna-hersavi*

80. Genius of inevitable knowing

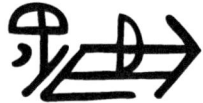

Angel – *Litple-savuhar*

81. Eliminating dependency through self-sovereignty

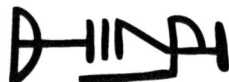

Angel – *Asva-nestavur*

82. Directionlessness through remembered wholeness

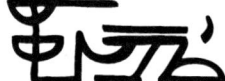

Angel – *Biriset-anu*

83. Knowing complete fullness in aloneness

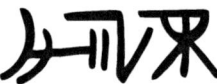

Angel – *Kivahet-eltravu*

84. Cutting the ties of inner relationships

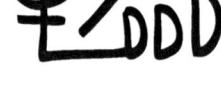

Angel – *Ekbar-retanu*

85. Replacing duty and responsibility with inevitable action

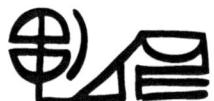

Angel – *Achvar-sihatre*

86. Removing inner dictators through perception

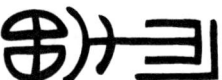

Angel – *Bispar-raktanu*

87. Balanced maturity through poise

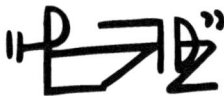

Angel – *Esvra-suhit-nanachva*

88. Graceful transitions through surrender

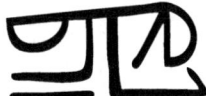

Angel – *Arektrava*

89. Dissolving the illusion of needing boundaries

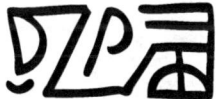

Angel – *Runanech-sitravi*

90. Minimizing friction through inevitable living

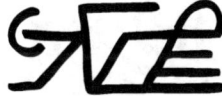

Angel – *Esklet-birasechvi*

91. Inner serenity through trust

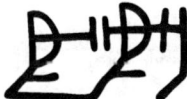

Angel – *Nesarut-paresta*

92. Pristineness of all dream states

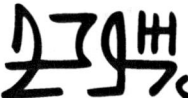

Angel – *Arsunat-achvetranu*

93. Responding to recognized intrinsic worth

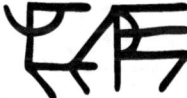

Angel – *Husaneck-spi-ura*

94. Uncompromising focus on the Infinite Being

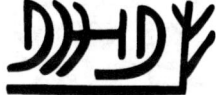

Angel – *Nensak-hesta-vrabit*

95. Purity in our physical environment

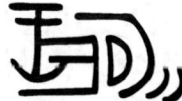

Angel – *Elklasut-manunech*

96. Knowing the eternal perfection of our body

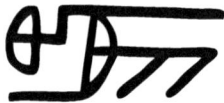

Angel – *Ritravit-asvanut*

97. Undifferentiated field

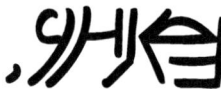

Angel – *Neksut-vilsavar*

101. Maturity of interpretation

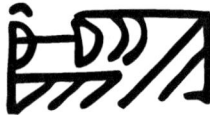

Angel – *Kiranat-minavu*

98. The fluid interplay of
chaos and order

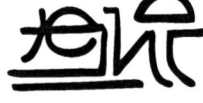

Angel – *Birapla-suknasut*

102. Refinement of responding to
authentic promptings

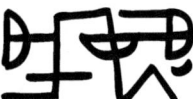

Angel – *Hasaklet-bisparu*

99. The high alchemy of
the 9th direction

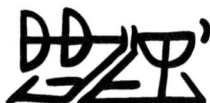

Angel – *Esba-pitre-aruk*

103. Integrity of all dream states

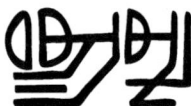

Angel – *Neksa-usbahur*

100. The release of guilt through
the release of worth

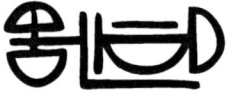

Angel – *Mechta-suhitvi*

104. Impeccable choices

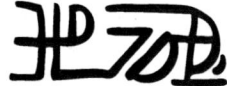

Angel – *Raksut-pliplesh-plaha*

105. Untainted dreaming

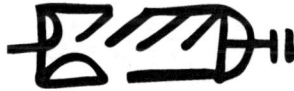

Angel – *Mesetu-renavik*

106. Self-sovereign journey through dream states

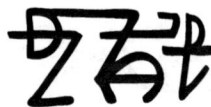

Angel – *Elseba-runahit*

107. Uncompromising expression

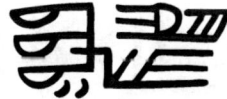

Angel – *Sihuklet-plisevar*

108. Faith in the seeming impossible

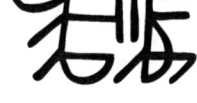

Angel – *Areknos-prusit*

109. Exponential fluid responsiveness

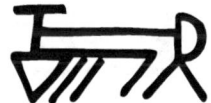

Angel – *Nenekstu-si-uter*

110. Creative solutions

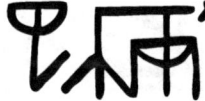

Angel – *Virspe-pletplehur*

111. Unquestionable faithfulness to the Infinite

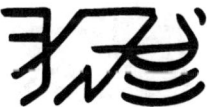

Angel – *Kirach-nanestu-uhar*

112. Releasing imprisoning beliefs

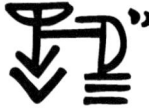

Angel – *Biret-arskla-varavit*

113. Fearless surrender and trust

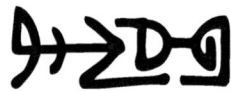

Angel – *Spubach-peresu*

117. Expressing fearless courage through perception

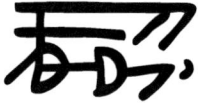

Angel – *Mishetu-nanskave*

114. The enjoyment of veils of mystery

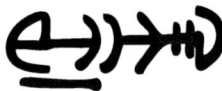

Angel – *Bliplaver-irastu*

118. Conscious wielding of the tools of the game

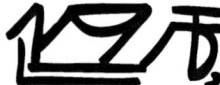

Angel – *Plisbatur-ures*

115. Engaged awareness through omniperspectives

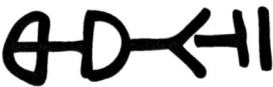

Angel – *Kiritna-vranave*

119. The freedom of the direction of through

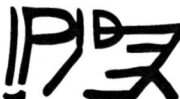

Angel – *Archbanus-skeleva*

116. Exposing unfathomable beauty

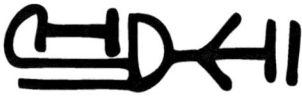

Angel – *Sutiranit-pireta*

120. Knowing unselfconscious virtuosity

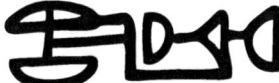

Angel – *Kelshanur-aras*

121. Freedom from the bondage of words

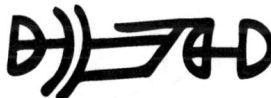

Angel – *Kirchbivatur*

122. Becoming the interpretative dancer

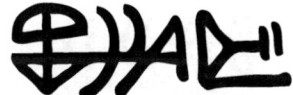

Angel – *Nensahit-areklava*

123. Surrender to the art of uncontrived expression

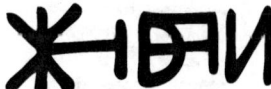

Angel – *Situnit-kirsava*

124. Immersal into the flow of Infinite Intent

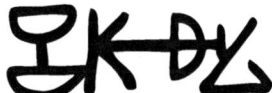

Angel – *Knechva-siter*

125. The integrated expression of chaos and order

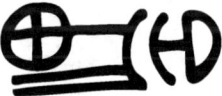

Angel – *Evarus-presprahet*

126. The equal value of opposites

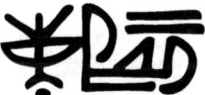

Angel – *Bliseter-sukvarut*

127. The removal of inner mirrors through the release of the tyranny of the heart

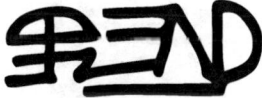

Angel – *Nekvrasut-brivabes*

128. Embracing the undefinable sweetness of life

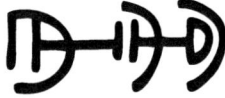

Angel – *Esech-nenesu*

129. Unlocking the fields
of mystery

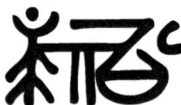

Angel – *Bisbarech-usetu*

130. Expressing limitless depth
of being

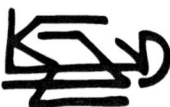

Angel – *Kiresat-pitrehus*

131. Exploring limitless width
of experience

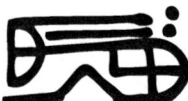

Angel – *Eskla-vibret-aranu*

132. Experiencing limitless fertile
possibilities

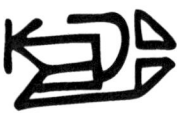

Angel – *Ekeva-suvatet*

133. Embraced vastness through
acknowledging the eternal self

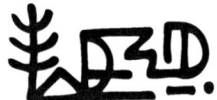

Angel – *Sikve-rutsavit*

134. Allowing the incomprehensible
to reveal itself

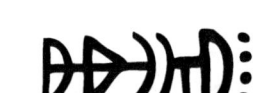

Angel – *Elsahut-mister*

135. Freedom from using mirrors
for guidance

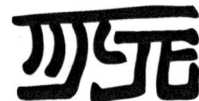

Angel – *Neneklu-brubaret*

136. Allowing the inspiration of
inconceivable excellence

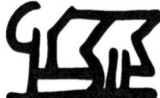

Angel – *Eratu-sikluhet*

137. Belief in the ability to move beyond preconceived boundaries

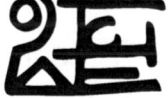

Angel – *Setvahit-esekla*

138. Fluid creations

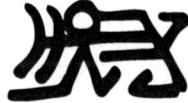

Angel – *Misetra-blibeset*

139. Releasing misalignments with Infinite Intent by dissolving expectations

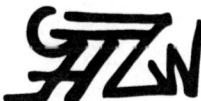

Angel – *Keratu-hiraset*

140. Releasing the need for uninspired entertainment

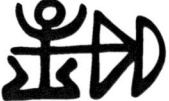

Angel – *Mireset-velesta*

141. Shelterless existence through uncompromised trust

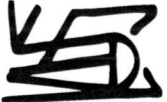

Angel – *Prakratu-subir*

142. Full interpretation of the 1,440 tones of the Calendar of Oneness

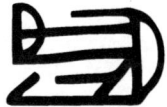

Angel – *Mileset-arsatu*

143. Living from the field of miracles

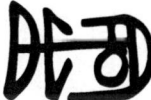

Angel – *Michbrevet-huraset*

144. Embodying all possibilities by becoming the Cosmic Alchemist

Ma-atma Suhat

Level II – Uruba-Satma

The Breaths of Timeless Regeneration

Secrets of the Whale Libraries

Secret 1
Eating

- Despise not your humanness as an unworthy vehicle of eternal expression. The functions of the body have sacred messages from the timeless expression of your being.
- Eat in silence, for the act of eating is a sacred communion with the natural kingdom. Through appreciation are you both fed by this experience. The plant and animal kingdom thrive through being appreciated.
- If the flesh of animals is eaten, the bowels need to be washed[2]. The toxic waste products of meat will else linger in the intestines for many years. This irrigation of the bowel needs to take place every 7 days if meat is consumed daily.
- Like the plucking of a string of a musical instrument, causing the strings of other instruments nearby to tremble in resonant sympathy, so too food affects you. It provides a note that causes certain notes within you to vibrate in a sympathetic response. This is the way nutrition stimulates the fullness of expression that produces health[3].
- Many remember the time of innocence when individuated life began and eating was not necessary, for resonance between beings served the same purpose – of reminding one another of songs that needed to be sung. As life explored density, more notes became unsung, and the ability to hear the notes of inspiration became lessened. Food became a way to stimulate unsung songs.

2 Enemas do not reach deeply enough. Colonics are far more effective.
3 This is also the way homeopathy works.

- The preferred way to eat is with your hands, for metal utensils disturb the song of the food[4]. If metal is used, let the handles be of the wood of trees. Let your ploughs be of copper; your pots be ceramic.

- Eat not standing up or lying down, nor when in stress, that the stomach be receptive to receive the food. Lie not immediately after eating, but if you must, let it be on your right side.

- Eat in silence as far as possible, that the communion with your food be deep and powerful. Pause in gratitude for the life you are ingesting, that the benefits may be increased one hundred fold. Eat your largest meal when the sun is high, and eat not after the sun has sunk below the horizon, that your body may rest in peace.

- Let your body become a grounding rod on Earth by balancing[5] your food and sitting on the ground every day. The neutral charge of such a one averts catastrophes and helps all in his environment flourish.

- Many seek to return to a self-sovereign state of having no need for sustenance. Freedom from the need for food can only come to the surrendered life in which the Infinite Song of Existence sings through your being. Only when you are authentically expressing shall you be free.

- Most avoid acknowledging the fullness of the present because they are so preoccupied with the past.

---

4 Homeopathy remedies too, should not come in contact with metal.
5 By 'balanced' diet to assist a neutral charge in the body, the records are referring to a balanced pH (alkaline/acid ratio) in the body. Too much starch or meat for instance would create an acidic body, prone to disease.
    The records specify the time required for either sitting or walking barefoot on the ground, as ' the time the sun would move the distance of two fingers, held at arm's length, through the sky.' This is roughly 45 to 60 minutes per day. Sitting on concrete would also work.

- We second-guess the fullness of the moment through judgement, thinking that something is lacking or imperfect. There is no failure – we have whatever is needed to contribute to the fullness of the moment. Judgement of what is lacking or the illusion that outcome could be failure is born of blindness. A grass stalk blowing in the wind cannot see that its movement is not just haphazard. From above, the sweeping dance of the field of grass as it is stroked by the wind can be seen in huge moving patterns. We lack the perspective of the grand scheme of things because of the limited ability of the egoic self to see.

Secret 2
Sacred Sexuality and Relationship

- Many programs there are, given by the tyrants of man, that deliberately create guilt of sexuality and shame of the body. The power of sexuality is so great that were it known, the tyrants would be tyrants no more.

- All beings have their magic, but man has lost his way. The magic of man can be restored by remembering the potency of sexuality and by evolving his concept of the expression and purpose of sexuality.

- Like the iceberg that lies mostly beneath the ocean, the true sexuality of humanity is largely unexpressed. When aspects are unexpressed, our eyes see life by what it lacks, rather than what it is. The more of ourselves we express, the more we are pleasantly amazed by what we encounter on our never-ending journey of existence.

- The feminine within all, holds the poetic perspective. See yourself through the eyes of the poet, for only then can you see another the same. Adorn your bodies and faces. Let your clothing reflect the song you wish to sing with your day, rather than to hide or shape the parts of your body you do not find acceptable. The body and clothing, and other adornments you may choose, are the joint poetic expression of your being.

- Sexuality is the holy communion within the temple of self-discovery you call relationship. Relationship is ignited by the spark of romantic attraction, but then tends to dwindle in its magical intensity. The linear progression of occurrences redefines it in ever-diminishing ways the more we label and think we know our partners. Like a sound that echoes back and forth, in decreasing magnitude between a canyon's walls, is the linear progression of a relationship.

- Think not you know another, for their vastness is beyond your comprehension. If their responses are predictable, they have been captured by the imagined prison bars of belief systems. The evolved sexual interaction with your partner can liberate through the depth of the experience.

- The gift of deeply aware sexuality is to change the linear progression of life, which results in aging or the dwindling of romance into mediocrity. Change comes like a series of starbursts that shatter the prisons of existing paradigms, rather than like a fading echo.

- Have no agenda, nor expected outcome, but the joyous communion of the real touching the real with your partner. For within each dwells that which is timeless presence. The desire for outcome stifles life's spontaneous song. From expectation comes linear mediocrity. From spontaneity comes orgasmic starbursts.

- The core grief of man is the inequity and discrepancy in how much is given and how little is received. Deep, evolved sexuality flushes up core griefs long buried, creating fear that when one expresses in fullness, the other may spiral into volatile insanity. But when the real beginningless core of one, seeks out the real in another, the dross of the past rises and is consumed by the fire, and blows away like ashes in the wind. In this way, change is leveraged beyond linear change.

- In mutual sexual surrender, man's obsession to know can be released as two become one. The songs yet unsung within each can be awakened. The song of innocent trust in playful adventure can take the place of planned strategy. The song of childlike wonderment at experiential discoveries of the self, takes the place of the obsession to know.

- Take time to enter the beauty of another and allow the other to access you by lowering your shields. Then shall your true essence meet that of another. Know that you each are a portal into infinity, through which you may enter with reverence. Then shall the pure notes of your being resonate in a fluid, harmonious symphony. You shall find, in the timeless moments of your union, that the outer and inner have become one, as you ricochet with each breath between the depths of your partner and yourself.

- Know the rapture of the orgasms of the body by knowing the orgasms of the soul. The intense appreciation of another's potency and attraction can be called gratitude – the core origin of an evolved physical orgasm. Deep love and inclusiveness is the origin of the peak experience known as an emotional climax. The latter can be experienced with another, or with an experience of oneness with nature or art.

- The third form of orgasm is of the spirit. It arises from peak states of praise and is often referred to as rapture. The body, soul and spirit are unreal vehicles of our experiences as we pass through life, death and ascension. These three types of orgasms burst the boundaries of their grip of illusion on our reality.

- Sing now with your lives the song of complete self-expression, that it may be remembered that these three mirrors that form the matrices of existence have never been separated. Then shall the indivisible, timeless form that has had no beginning, lift you beyond the treadmill of the illusional journey of life, death and ascension, to the miracle of eternal, ever-renewed form.

- When sexuality is denied as unworthy or unholy, sexual tension often is redirected into activity. This increases electricity in the body, making sexual expression more mechanical and perfunctory, while reducing the magic sexuality can bring.

- When the balanced, grounded polarity that evolved sexuality can bring is not present, the hyper-electric charge of the body calls in catastrophic change rather than graceful transition. A balanced polarity of a person creates a grounding rod that helps the seeds of potential in others flourish. We stimulate fullness of expression in others by living it ourselves.

> *Chevevech nesetuch hurasvavi menevash asti kravis.*
> Authentic expression eliminates mirrored divisions.

> *Keresech prihas nanasvi uresta blavabit eres*
> *kerenat spihur mesenech krihavi.*
> The sense of adventure stimulates open receptivity
> to the wonder of self-discovery.

> *Prihas usetve minach usevi krivanut plihavas*
> *krives ereh eseta mesenech uset harasvi.*
> Contracted and shallow perspectives destroy the poetic
> perspective necessary for refined expression.

Secret 3
Abundant and Authentic Living

Kishat ararech minetvi huraras kilechba husanet
echparurarek esetvi manunach petreve skluharu-bat.
Innocence is not blindness, but comes from deeper
vision that sees the eternal within the heart of illusion.

- Our core fears seek resolution and obstruct the effortless flow
of the divine expressing through us. A prominent fear is lack of
abundance. Abundance is enhanced by praise and gratitude.

Spererech nispa arurat misenech vribasbi huret vrispechva
misurut kletvavi.
Praise is an exalted state of being that lives above appearances
and acknowledges the fullness of the moment.

- Soul, body and spirit are the vehicles of illusion that are formed
from the stories and identities of the past. They deliberately create
trigger events that bring back issues from the past in order to
strengthen their existence by our repeating these former events.
As we become aware of events influencing us from the past, view
them briefly from a perspective of yourself as vast as the cosmos,
and then shift your focus to the fullness of the moment. Like the
stalk of grass blowing in the wind, know the perfections of the
large picture manifesting through its parts, even if it cannot be
seen.

- What then can the desires of your heart seek that is not already
there? What prayers can you offer to heal the imagined lack of the
moment? The desires that you feel are but the stirrings that awaken
the unfolding notes of the Song of the Self.

- The folly of others has been a source of fear – those who in a lower reality dwell – for they seem to be the many, and you are but one. Could they not bring the cloak of density and its consequences into your reality? Know now with compassion that the misbehavior of another is but an expression of their eternal luminosity reaching for its place upon the imagined stage of existence.

- The reality of each being is a unique slice of existence, and in that slice which contains all representations of the whole, he is the sovereign point of origin. When he is at one with the expression of the whole, his reality will be one of grace. When he closes himself to the gentle whisperings of his eternal being, and tries to impose his agenda onto his environment, his world becomes a cage in which he must wrestle with the demons of his own fear. Another's reality cannot affect him – two different slices are they. All that he can ever know is that all that in his slice of reality, can be effected by him.

- The world we know must change as we do, for in the spaceless space of eternity, we dwell within all and all dwells within us. We are not limited by numbers, since division is but an imaginary tool of the poetic expression of our being. Release now the fear that your endeavors cannot have the significant impact you intend.

- The guidance we seek from within or without, affirms relationship and strengthens division. The mirrors of the external exist also in the internal when we differentiate between the inner and outer. We are the portal of spacelessness; seek not the answers without nor within, but let the emotional nuances within and subtle currents without, guide your attitudes. From these shall the qualities of the day, through the attitudes they evoke, steer the inevitable and right action of your life.

- From the food that you choose, or the sexual images that arise, you are reminded of the songs you have forgotten. To the aware, they stimulate the emotions and the attitudes that are dormant, to bring new expression to your life. View nutrition not as a need, but an inspiration.

- The mirrors of body, soul and spirit have become the identities we think we are. But they are the garments we clothe ourselves in, for like all garments, they are a means to artistic expression, fashioned from the stories we have created. When we think that our form will perish if we discard them, we hold onto them until they become our armor. But the fluid form we are has eternally been.

- True eternal form is beyond the matter you know. It is that which has worn matter like a garment. Within eternal form, soul and spirit are aspects inseparably expressing as one with matter. There are belief systems that cast the separate shadows of the divided expressions of body, soul and spirit.

- The separating beliefs are:
  (1) That the realm of soul promises freedom after death from the constrictions of physicality. Soul promises freedom but does not allow individuality of expression.
  (2) False values have been placed on the levels of soul (death) and spirit (ascension). They are thought to be more holy, merciful and knowing than the physical.
  (3) The physical has been seen to be more mundane and mediocre. But to the one that is aware, its stark contrasts (causing the tension that maintains its density) offer the most exquisite poetry and deepest rapture.

- Abundance is the triumph over the illusion of limitation, the song of power over appearances. Refuse to accept programs of negativity. Minimize lack by shifting the focus: envision the opposite of what you fear. Live abundantly in your own reality and all else shall flourish.

Bereshpa mishet harusta misech haras erestatve.
There is not adversity, only reminders of unsung songs.

I Am

I am the thunderous clamor
Of one thousand pounding drums,
Heralding to an astounded world
The eternal glory of the rising sun.

I am the elusive, unfathomable silent wonder
Of a rose unfurling the mantle of its velvet petals
In the heart of the night.

I am the ever-receding depth of darkness of the starry sky,
Offering its shrine to the shining celestial jewels
Of the still whispering constellations.

I am the wild laughter of the thunder,
And the burning embrace of the lightning,
Piercing the sky in an outburst of joy
Across a summer storm.

Eternal mystery am I,
Revealing myself through riddles
Throughout the fabric of time and space,
Relentlessly weaving ever-changing scenes
On the dreamed canvas of my existence.

Marc, Belgium

Secret 4
The Nature of Change

- The nature of change can be either cataclysmic, or a graceful metamorphosis from one level of existence to another. Cataclysmic change comes from the surface and forces us into re-evaluation and the eventual adjustment of core beliefs.

- Graceful change is precipitated by a deep and profound shift of core attitudes and beliefs. This foundational adjustment filters into the surface experiences of everyday life, resulting in graceful and supported change.

- The future is written in the moment, in the same way the past is fluidly reformed by a well-lived moment. If we abandon the moment by fearing or anticipating the future, we forfeit the priceless gift of the power of the moment. We lose the ability to not only determine the quality of our existence, but the way in which change will occur – with grace or cataclysmically.

- We are standing on the cusp of a deep core shift in cosmic and planetary existence. This will most certainly filter through into the surface conditions of everyday life. Whether we experience these changes with grace or trauma depends on how fluidly we can synchronize our deep, inner change with the profound and fundamental changes taking place at the heart of existence.

- We have been part of linear change as a way of life for eons of existence – this is about to change. Linear change causes deterioration in all circumstances, unless we constantly feed it energy to maintain ideal conditions. This principle is called inertia.

- The peak condition of the body, or a relationship for instance, deteriorates without constant efforts of renewal. Linear change is like an echo bouncing off canyon walls – it becomes weaker every time it changes direction. The canyon walls can be equated to cataclysmic change that forces life into a different direction. Cataclysms cause shock, and shock lowers consciousness by creating a loss of life force and energy.

- The way life changes, from one expression to the next throughout the cosmos, will become a starburst rather than a line bouncing off the membranes or matrices of space.

- The movement of life within a confined space is the experience of linear time. The space is formed by limiting belief systems that confine our experiences within matrices.

- The effect of exponential starburst changes at the heart of life, is the shattering of layers of matrices. This changes not only the way time will be experienced, but also effects instant freedom from old belief systems.

- Previously changes came from cataclysms and opposition (the canyon walls). The result was deterioration in the quality of life. The changes at the heart of existence will now come from rapture, and will release profound energy and life force (supported change) to the surface conditions of everyday life.

- As the cosmos transcends the principle of inertia, one of the core griefs of man can be healed: the belief that our output (effort) always exceeds our input (rewards). It is now possible to flourish and to achieve results more effortlessly – embrace this belief. Replace doubt with glad expectations. Repeat the daily affirmation: *I flourish by releasing old expectations.*

- As the gap between cause and effect closes, thought and feelings will more rapidly manifest. Be aware of your fears, but immediately redirect your attention to their opposite manifestation: If you fear lack of resources, acknowledge your fear, but immediately pour energy into the visualization of abundance coming into your life until what you fear seems unreal. Do not pretend negative emotions are not there, as one strengthens what one opposes, but rather withhold your energy from them by redirecting it elsewhere.

- Live with deep awareness. Slow life down and take a few pauses in your daily activities to appreciate deeply your environment, others, your many blessings and the Earth. Gratitude brings increase and self-appreciation. By allowing yourself to be inspired by your environment, you life becomes revitalized.

- Attuning to the unfolding core of existence through gratitude, love and praise, creates peak orgasmic experiences of the body (sexuality with the self or another), the soul (emotional rapture such as that inspired by art, music or deep love) and the spirit (through praise resulting from the recognition of the perfection unfolding beyond the appearances). These create starburst experiences that shatter old matrices and birth new possibilities.

Secret 5
Nuances of Eternal Expression

Ten fears are there, that cause victimization. Ten feelings that move with silent power from our eternal core, that when expressed, can remove these fears. Self-pity becomes replaced by the fullness of our eternal song.

The Fears of Victimization
1. Fear of victimization from authority
2. Fear of the folly of others
3. Fear of the tyranny of the body
4. Fear of the dictatorship of the soul
5. Fear of the control of the spirit
6. Fear of ancestral programs and heritage
7. Fear of insurmountable opposition
8. Fear of annihilation (not being worthy of life)
9. Fear of not being prepared or adequate (performance angst)
10. Fear of being unsupported

Nuances of Eternal Expression
1. Timeless self-sovereignty: Living from outside the matrix, one can direct, through slight intent, the experience within the matrix.
2. Receptive expression: Receiving inspiration from the world around us allows our expression to be aligned with unfolding existence.
3. Full appreciation through an omniperspective: We cannot find the inspiration from our environment by just using our eyes or ears alone. Allow yourself to absorb the eternal aspect of what you observe, feeling it through the inner as well as the outer senses.

4. Exponential discoveries: Change linear becoming to starburst, exponential becoming by leaving the past stories behind. Discard all identities. Allow the rapture of deep experience to shatter the shields of shallow vision.

5. Inspired Oneness: In seeing the beauty at the heart of all life, we awaken it in our own through resonance.

6. Unconditional love in response to recognition of beauty: Love evoked by inspiration is unconditional and without agenda. This transcends one of the biggest obstacles of the heart – loving without pain.

7. Truth as spontaneous expression of your eternal being: Truth cannot be sought, but needs to express as the free, pure spontaneity of your eternal self.

8. Awakening the eternal song by finding astonishing wonderment everywhere: We change our reality by seeking the poetry of our existence. By being aware of brutal circumstances, but choosing to focus on the praiseworthy, we empower a higher reality, benefitting all life.

9. Revitalizing communion with the timeless aspects in all things, through aware acknowledgment: Decay occurs by focusing on the imperfection of appearances. Life is revitalized by living from core to core through awareness.

10. Exchanging the mirrored existence for authentic expression: The five senses alone provide false information and trick us into thinking we know. A life of authentic expression acknowledges that, since life is forever new, nothing can be known. The truth of the moment must be felt.

The Perceptions of the Breaths
Freedom from the Ties that Bind

Timeless regeneration is the natural state of all individuated life forms. Constant renewal is only inhibited by the self-made bondage of our existence.

Identifying the etheric cords we have permitted to bind us and eliminating the root causes, permits timeless regeneration to take place. The breaths are designed to facilitate the removal of those cords, combined with the use of a power source and a 'cutting' wheel.

Some indigenous cultures have recognized that binding ties, caused by emotional needs and belief systems, as well as instinctual survival programs, erode the emotional, and eventually the physical bodies of humanity. They have used blue heron and eagle feathers to cut them, and tones and rattles to break up the areas of stagnation caused by them. This ensured the health of tribal members by allowing natural healing through self-regeneration to take place.

The Cords and How They Erode the Fields

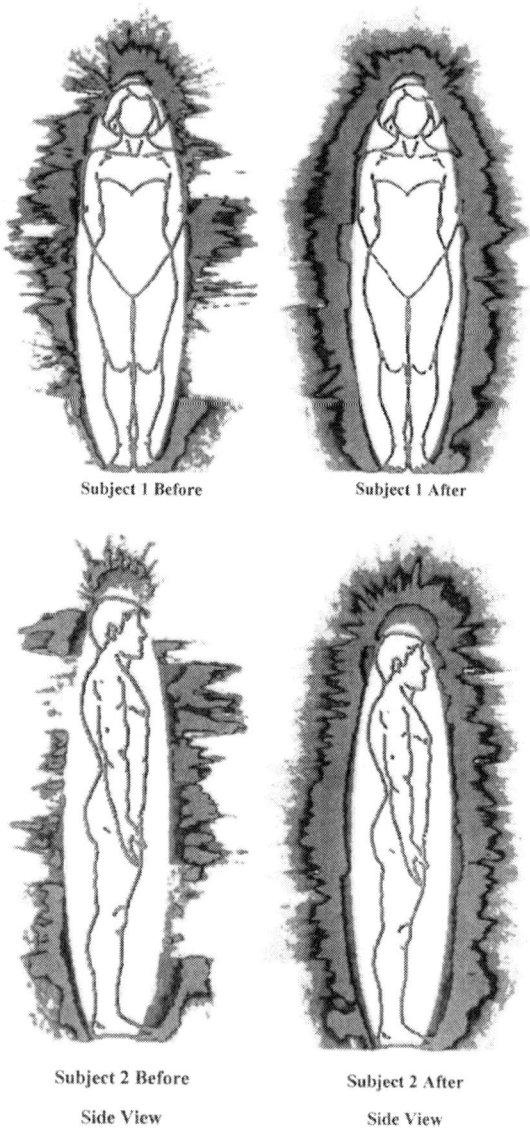

These images show the effect that cords can have on the fields around the body. The second image demonstrates changes / improvements to the field following a healing session by Almine.

The 18 Ties that Bind

Self-pity

1. Fear of disruption of destiny
2. Protectiveness against victimization
3. Programs of survival
4. Guilt over past choices
5. Blame for conduct of others
6. Fear of deprivation

Self-importance

1. Ties of obligation
2. Ties of the desire to fix
3. Belief systems of responsibility
4. Self-abandonment to serve others
5. Becoming captive of our strong suits
6. Defining oneself by past achievement

Self-reflection

1. Ties of the desire to improve
2. Ties of entitlement
3. Subservience to the arrogance of others
4. Accepting worldly standards
5. The bondage of belief in the law of compensation
6. Desires to pacify others for acceptance and peace

The Equation for Timeless Regeneration

Freedom from movement and measure

+

Freedom from the bondage of opposites

+

Freedom from inclusiveness and exclusiveness

+

Freedom from the fear of disruption of density

=

Revealed access to Timeless Regeneration

Uruba-Satma

The Breaths of Timeless Regeneration

*Beyond youth and aging, lies the
eternally renewed expression of transient
timelessness. To seek youth, is to promote
age. The result of flourishing through love,
praise, gratitude and trust is regeneration.*

The Breathing Technique of Uruba-Satma

Note: Prior to doing the Uruba-Satma Breaths, it is important that you have completed all 3 Levels of the Arasatma Breaths, the Nevi-Satma, the Twelve Breaths of Proxy and Level I of Ma-atma Suhat – the Sa-huna Satma Breaths. The Sa-huna Satma Breaths should be practiced at least once, followed by a day's break, before doing the Uruba-Satma Breaths.

To reduce the effects of detoxification on the body following these breath exercises, it is advisable that you have a day of rest and drink plenty of water.

The Wheels of Uruba-Satma:

- Create a stack of the 4 wheels to place below the feet. Place them in the following order:

  At the bottom place Wheel 4 – *The Wheel of Infinite Potential*
  On top of that place Wheel 3 – *The Formula of Boundlessness*
  Next place Wheel 2 – *The Wheel to Cut the Ties That Bind*
  On top place Wheel 1 – *The New Cosmic Template*

- As you lie comfortably on the floor, or a bed or massage table, the stack of 4 wheels will be at your feet. The wheels can be laminated for repeated use.

The Perceptions:

- Before each set of two in-and out-breaths, take several minutes to read and understand the perception and if necessary, release the cords found in your life.
- The diligence of doing this step enables the wheels to move through your body with ease. If a concept is not properly embodied and understood, a rotating wheel could get stuck. This will feel like

an uncomfortable pressure building up (often in the knees, neck, head, etc.). Release the pressure by pretending that there is a little mouth in the area and breathing out through it or by using more pressure to suck the wheels up with breath.

The Breaths:
* There are 24 in-and out-breaths and 12 perceptions to release bondage.
* Two in- and out-breaths accompany each perception.
* The 24 breaths are identical and each consists of a long, deep breath in, which sucks the wheels up from the feet, through the body. This is followed by a long, slow out-breath after they have moved out through the head.

Using the Breath with the Perceptions:
* First In-breath and Out-breath.
  Having contemplated the first perception, the top wheel will be envisioned as rotating clockwise and moving up through the body, followed closely by the second wheel from the top. Envision these two wheels moving up and out of the top of the head at the end of the first in-breath. As you draw the wheels up through the body, only focus on the rotating wheels and the breath and not the perception. Release the breath in a long, slow exhale, while at the same time emptying the mind.

* Second In-breath and Out-breath.
  For the next in-breath of the perception you are working with, envision the two remaining wheels following each other as they rotate clockwise up and out of the top of the head. Again focus on the rotating wheels and the breath and not the perception. Release the breath in a long, slow exhale, while at the same time emptying the mind.

- Continue until all 24 breaths and 12 concepts are completed.
  Repeat the pattern for all 12 perceptions, using Wheels 1 and 2 for
  Perceptions 3, 5, 7, 9 and 11 and Wheels 3 and 4 for Perceptions 4,
  6, 8, 10 and 12.

The Wheels of the
Uruba-Satma Breaths

Wheel I
The New Cosmic Template

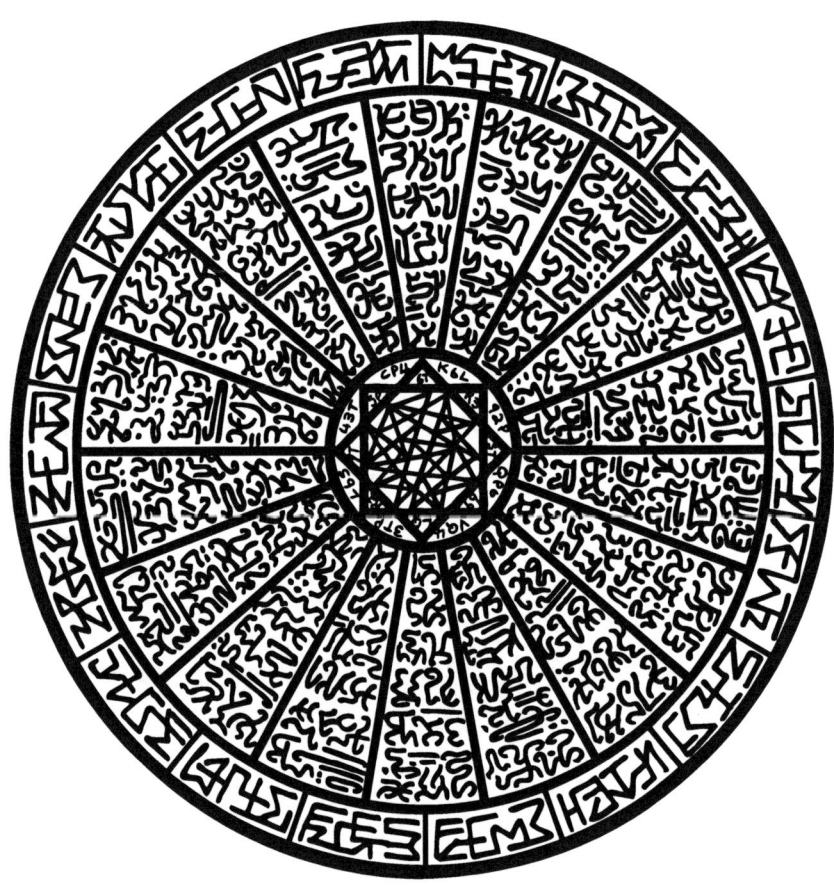

Menenech Usatvi Eres Harsatu Nunas
From evolved man let all be uplifted

Wheel 2
The Wheel to Cut the Ties That Bind

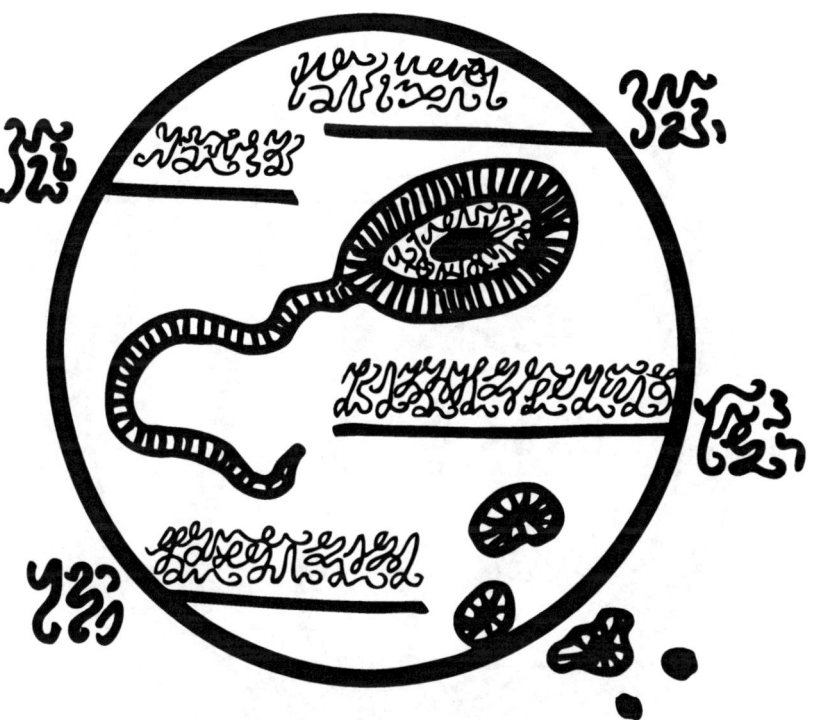

Nutrach ures paharasbi misetech manes
Cut now the ties of self-made bondage

Wheel 3

The Formula of Boundlessness

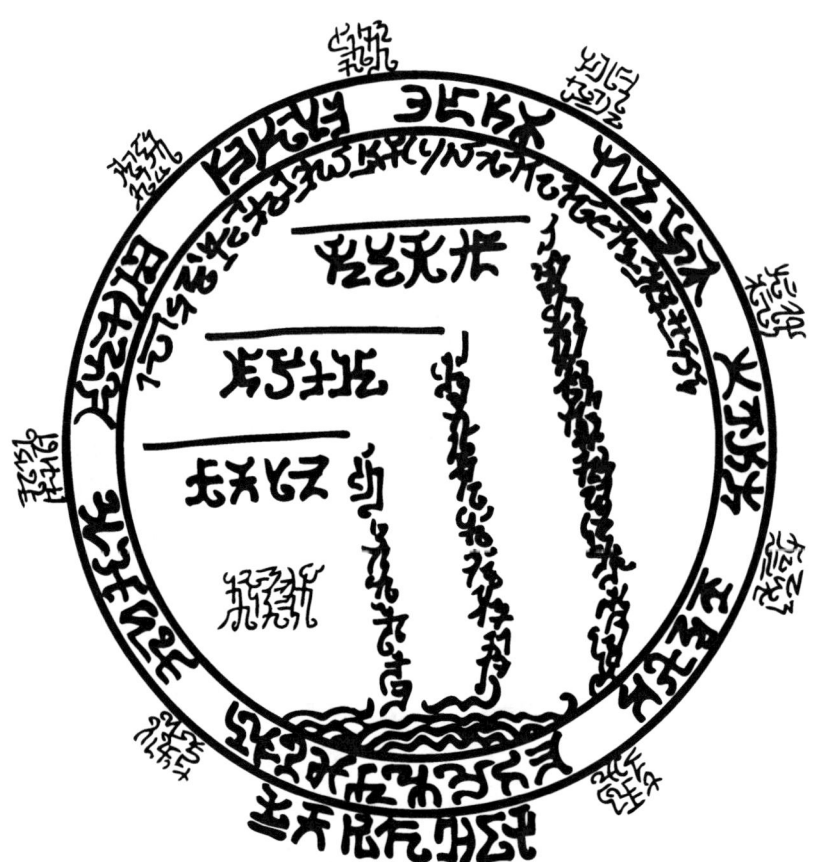

Shavech Virsata Manunesh Ashantavi
Sovereignty to the One Expressing as the Many

Wheel 4

The Wheel of Infinite Potential

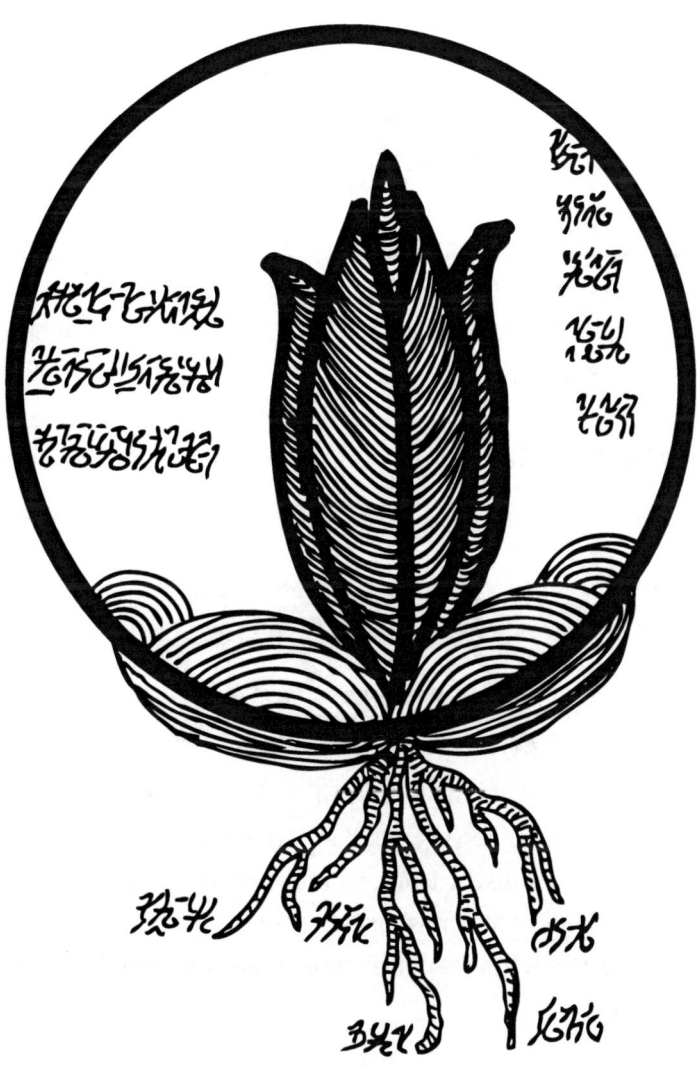

The 12 Perceptions of the Breaths
of Uruba-Satma

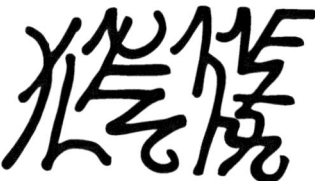

1. There are 18 basic fears, needs and belief systems that form the cords that bind us to the old bondage of the matrix of linear time. They can be divided into categories of self-pity, self-importance and self-reflection.

Affirmation: I dissolve self-pity, self-importance, and self-reflection.

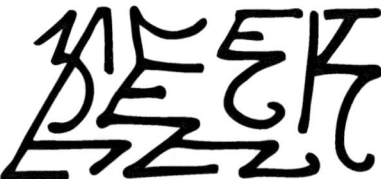

2. The separation from the feeling of being one with Source came from a contracted perspective that formed the egoic self. This was caused by a discordant tone in the cosmos: ingratitude. An individuation saw itself as far less than the Embodiment of the Infinite and a feeling of deprivation arose. Ingratitude for gifts followed.

Affirmation: I embrace life in gratitude.

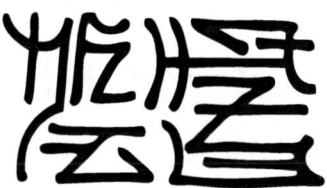

3. The pain of alienation caused a feeling of aloneness and loss. This caused separate life forms to seek tribes for comfort and security, the way a newborn seeks comfort and security by making a tribe with its mother. We try to equalize others to form a tribe. The tribe tries to pull down those who excel. Those who excel try and lift the tribe.

Affirmation: I see the perfection in all levels of expression.

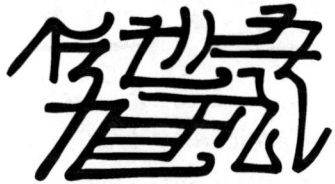

4. Tribes support only as a reward for letting them control the individual. The pain of bondage replaces the pain of aloneness. Self-abandonment in favor of the service to the tribe takes place. The pain of alienation from Source becomes compounded by alienation from ourselves.

Affirmation: I live authentically in full self-expression.

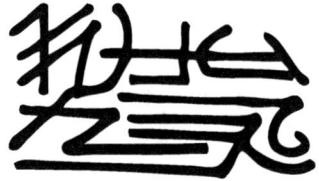

5. The pain of alienation and suppression caused the dialogue of the mind to form, keeping us out of the heart and in the mind. The dialogue of the mind is formed by resistance to life and keeps us in bondage of linear time. The dialogue of the mind keeps us out of the moment where we are in touch with our feelings, by reflecting on the moment gone by or anticipating the moment to come.

Affirmation: I live in the moment by being in surrendered trust.

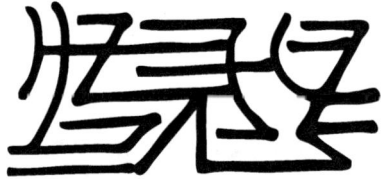

6. Self-abandonment, by not accessing our feelings or not expressing authentically, brings addiction. Addiction to tension arises. Tension levels dictate the levels of density in the bodies of all beings. The denser the body, the more energy is required to sustain it and the more it is subject to sickness and pain. This creates further ingratitude for the gifts of life by drawing our attention to discomforts. Pain in a less dense body is experienced as pressure.

Affirmation: I release the density caused by inner tension through acknowledging the perfection of my experience.

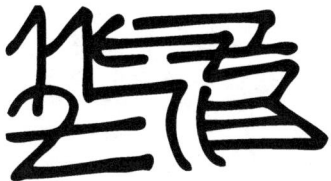

7. We step off the treadmill of cords and bondage by being home for ourselves and putting things we enjoy in every day, and learning to turn duties into acts of praise and devotion. We express fully that which makes our hearts sing with the confidence that what is good for us is ultimately good for all.

Affirmation: I find as many things to be grateful for each day as I possibly can, and allow them to inspire me with love for life.

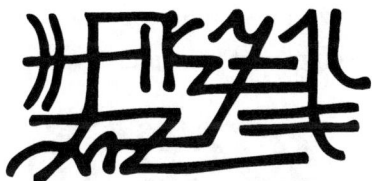

8. Fun as contrived enjoyment is a concept that belongs to the old matrix. Wayshowers that leave the matrix behind for a life of higher consciousness must evolve this concept. When we separate enjoyment out from the rest of our daily activities, they become joyless and then become a cause for resentment. It is in enjoying all areas of our lives by living with our hearts open, that everything becomes fun.

Affirmation: Enjoyment permeates all I do, removing the boundaries between fun and work.

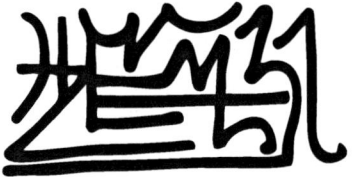

9. It is the self-abandoning attitude that believes that we are the ones responsible for the enjoyment of others: that we are needed to please those who come into our homes, our presence, or our lives. This living for others' wellbeing, deprives us of our own wellbeing and enjoyment. The living for others at the cost of ourselves, is the primary cause of cancer. Being fully present for ourselves, creates the natural warmth towards others that has no agenda and no need to entertain others.

Affirmation: I recognize the validity of others' tears and allow them their sorrow as a chosen part of their journey.

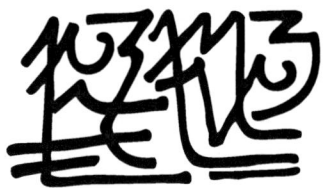

10. When the inner feminine seeks to create a pleasant quality of life for others (the feminine is that which concerns itself with quality versus quantity), while abandoning her own joy, she loses touch with her own femininity. She becomes masculine in that she loses herself in proactivity (+) rather than receptivity (–), which is feminine. The societal program is that a woman's worth is measured by how much she can give.

Affirmation: My inner feminine is open to receiving the bounty and gifts of the moment. My life unfolds with grace.

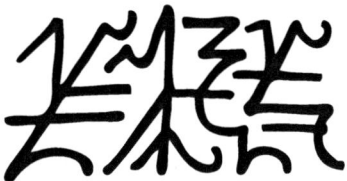

11. Life's unfolding change is unavoidable. When we keep trying to improve the journey's quality for others, we interfere with their growth and development. This prohibits change from taking place with grace and creates hardship for them through forced change. When we do what is right for ourselves, we are living our highest truth, and we automatically do what is right for another.

Affirmation: My gift to others is my full presence. From being home for myself, I radiate warmth to all.

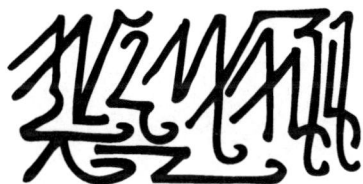

12. Enjoyment comes from the next inevitable step: the right step taken in clarity, not from what the world's programs tell us is enjoyable. When we are busy assessing how other people are feeling or trying to control their level of enjoyment, we cannot find the promptings from within to tell us what the next step of the dance of life is that will bring us joy.

Affirmation: In the quietness of surrendered trust and the confidence of the benevolence of my being, I dwell in my strength.

Closing

The release of guilt and cords that tie us to others and the past, requires what the ancient mystics call 'eagle vision' – to hover above the situation or relationship that has captured you and view it with detached, non-judgmental discernment. Gain the insights and assess what and where you have to let go.[6]

Write a letter to give, or not to give, to another with compassion, firmness and clarity if necessary. State what insights and understanding you have gained that have given you compassion, but also which areas of the relationship are not acceptable. If you believe you want to continue the relationship, state what changes you will make in your conduct to prevent getting roped into dysfunctional interaction.

6 See Appendix I – How to Access Past Events and Relationships

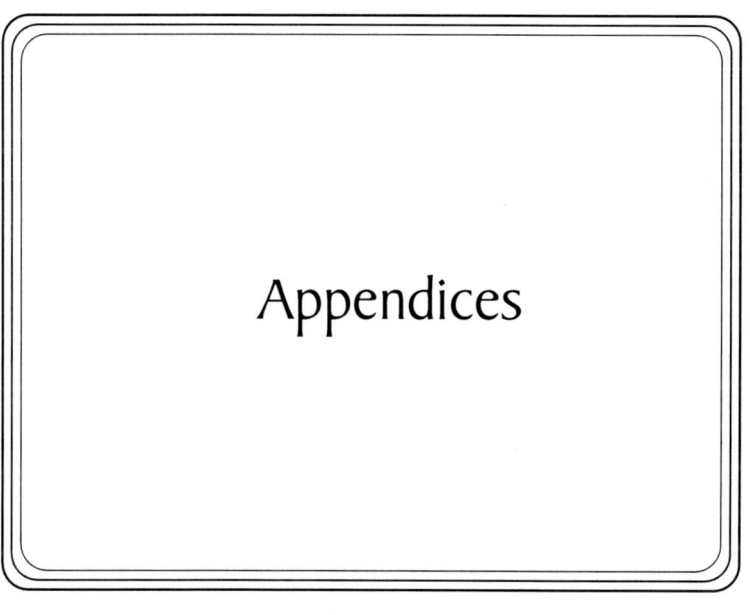

Appendices

Appendix I

How to Assess Past Events and Relationships

Excerpt from *Journey to the Heart of God*

1. What is the lesson? Look for the lesson that our higher self wishes us to embrace. For example, the lesson may be that we need to speak our truth. It could manifest as laryngitis, or someone may appear to mirror to us that we frequently suppress our voice. He or she may violate our boundaries to get our attention. We need to protect ourselves by voicing our truth that this behavior is unacceptable. Accepting the unacceptable is not saintly, it is dysfunctional.

2. What is the contract? Everyone who interacts with us has made an agreement prior to this incarnation to assist with our growth and for us to assist in theirs. They may have agreed to push us over the edge, and we may do likewise for them. Ask, "What is the contract we are playing out?" It is with great love that many agreed while in the spirit world to be our catalysts. When we are in perfect equilibrium, there is no growth so it is a signal to the universe to knock us off balance so the lessons may continue. Thus we pull relationships into our lives that test us in every way imaginable.

3. What is the role? Am I playing the victim? Am I playing the teacher or the student? What role am I playing within this contract? Also look at the role the other person is playing. For example, we may have a tyrant in our life. It may be our spouse, mother, or boss. Once you establish that, see who you are in relation to that person's role. Remember, we may change our role at any time because we create our reality.

4. What is the mirror? We pull relationships into our life that mirror one of the following things: an aspect of who we are, what we have given away, what we still place judgment on, or what we haven't developed yet. For example, if our innocence is gone, we may find ourselves intensely attracted to a young person. If we have given our integrity away, we might fall in love with a missionary who, in our eyes, represents integrity. Another thing that can be mirrored is that which we judge. If we have problems dealing with people who lie, then we are judging them and therefore attract liars.

5. What is the gift? Every person we encounter has come to give us a gift and receive one as well. This applies even with the most casual acquaintance. Ask, "What gift am I supposed to give this person?" It may be something as simple as offering him the gift of unconditional love, or we may recognize something beautiful in him that nobody else has seen. We may genuinely listen to someone and for the first time in years, they feel heard and understood. (Note: The last four questions deal with our attitudes surrounding the answers to the first five questions)

6. Can I allow? This is the point of discerning what has to be allowed, what has to be changed, and finding the courage to act. Imagine yourself as the water in a river. If a rock is in front of you, should you oppose it or flow around the rock? We have masterfully created every situation in our life, even the rock. Is this a test of flexibility and surrender? Or is this a battle for us to fight? A battle is only worth fighting if the stakes are worth winning. If you have already learned the lesson, no need to refight this battle.

7. Can I accept? We cannot accept the painful things that happen to us unless we begin to see the perfection underlying the web of appearances. A common belief is that we were placed on the wheel of reincarnation, suffering lifetime after lifetime, until we

have lived enough lives to become perfect. We have been created perfectly with the ability to be a creator. Thoughts combined with emotions create our environment. The heart is like a microphone: the stronger the emotions, the stronger the universe's response to manifest our desires. But the universe doesn't discriminate, it will manifest whatever we think – positive or negative. It is important that we accept that we have co-created the situation, which removes any feelings of having things done 'to' us.

8. Can I release? To release is to let go of the energy surrounding the person or event. If we don't release, we keep it alive by feeding it energy through thoughts (sometimes subconsciously). Even if someone has violated us in some way, working through these steps to gain the larger insights behind the appearances, changes the focus to an eternal perspective. It reveals the perfection underlying the appearances.

9. Can I be grateful? If we have gone through the previous eight steps and can feel true gratitude for the insights gained, it raises consciousness. Gratitude is a powerful attitude that can assist us to transfigure into a higher state of being. It changes stumbling blocks into stepping stones. If we have completed the first eight steps and don't feel gratitude, going through them again to gain even deeper insights will help.

The prize for cutting the ties that bind of guilt, fear, pain, anger and protectiveness, is nothing short of the ultimate freedom from the treadmill of human games and dysfunctionality. The games are acts of resistance to life and this further traps us in linear time and cycles of life and death. The breaths and accompanying self-examination and perceptions are therefore also designed to set us free from linear time. Releasing resistance to life makes limitless resources available to us. Coupled with freedom from the ravages of linear time, the mastery of these techniques can produce an eternally renewing existence: the sacred purpose of Arasatma, the Breaths of Eternal Life.

Appendix II

Symbols Versus Sigils

To understand sigils, we must first understand what symbols entail. We will also need to know the meanings of sigils in order to properly understand and utilize them as they are given later in this book.

A symbol represents something, whereas a sigil describes something. When someone sees a BMW or a Mercedes symbol, it represents upper middle-class vehicles of quality and distinction. On the other hand, the symbol for a Rolls Royce or Bentley represents elite vehicles that speak of a privileged lifestyle of dignity and wealth.

So much is deduced just from one symbol. A Rolls Royce evokes images of walled estates, chauffeurs, enough and accustomed money, as opposed to the symbol of a Ferrari which speaks of more flamboyant taste.

Whereas symbols are common in our everyday world, the use of sigils is virtually forgotten. Even in mystery schools, their hidden knowledge eludes most mystics. But throughout the cosmos all beings of expanded awareness utilize sigils and only a few left-brain-oriented races use symbols and those primarily in alphabets.

The reason is this: If we use the word 'LOVE', we have combined four symbols (letters representing certain sounds) to make one symbol (the word that represents a feeling). But love is one of the building blocks of the cosmos, like space or energy.[7] It can also represent many different nuances within the emotion of love (which is the desire to include) and many other forms of dysfunctionality and degrees of need we mistakenly call 'love'.

---

7 Discussed in *Journey to the Heart of God,* The True Nature of the Seven Directions.

As we can see, the symbol or word can be very misleading since what it represents to one may not be what it represents to another. The sigil for love describes the quality or frequency of what is meant. It maps out the exact frequency of the emotion.

The sigil for someone's name would do the same. As the person or being rises in frequency, the sigil will change to reflect that. In the case of angels, even their names change. That is why the angel names or the goddess names have changed as the cosmos and Earth have ascended to a much higher frequency. In these higher realms the languages are different and reflect the higher frequencies.

When a person has accomplished a major task within the cosmos pertaining to the agreement they made with the Infinite, they also receive a 'meaning' with its accompanying sigil. When a being is called to do a task meant for the highest good, that being will come if you have its name and meaning. The being absolutely must come if, in addition, you have the sigil for the name and meaning.

Having someone's sigil is like having that person's phone number. Sigils not only describe what they represent, but are a means to communicate with what they represent.

Appendix III

The Seer Almine Answers Questions on the Arasatma Breaths

Q. Breath 1 refers to the *Lion's Gate*. What and where is this gate?

A. The translation of the name is *Atma* (breath) *seba* (lion's) *uhut* (gate). The Lion's Gate is the pineal gland. One of its main purposes is to clear the trigger events that bring old patterns and behavior back. These are held in the amygdala and the medulla holds the memories.

Q. Sometimes when I do these breaths, I feel resistance to moving the eyes. Is there a reason for this?

A. Many of the movements of the breath may feel like they should be done in the opposite way. For example, as you move the breath up the back of the skull, it doesn't feel as though your eyes should look up. This is because it is going through thresholds and breaking up old blockages. It is therefore important that you follow the directions as given.

Q. Breath 2 is called *The Breath of the Winged Ones,* why is this?

A. It is named so because it deals with blocks in self-expression. When our wings are clipped, we cannot fly. We cannot flourish when we have blocks to self-expression.

Q. The aphorism for Breath 2, Level I states: *"I am in surrendered stillness during automatic, proactive expression."* Can you explain this further?

A. What it means is that your actions are inevitable and automatic. It is action within rest. So at no time does it really require tension for the action to occur.

As you are working with your subconscious mind while doing these breaths, the aphorisms are more likely to be retained than if you were repeating them a hundred times without the breaths. For this reason it is really important that you hold an image of the meaning of them.

Q. I seem to be yawning as I do these exercises, why would this be?
A. Yawning is a sign of the movement of energy.

Q. The technique for Breath 2 states that the ribcage moves from right to left, and that it is important that this movement is isolated from rest of the body, with no movement of the rest of the body including the head, shoulders, abdomen and hips. Is there a specific reason for this?
A. The trachea lies between the lungs and it is in the trachea that a tremendous amount of density is held. Fears held in the trachea include the *fear that you can't breathe when you are coming through the birth canal* and *fear that you can't breathe during death.* Moving the ribcage fully from one side to the other on the out-breath moves the trachea and enables the trauma that is held there to be expelled.

Q. What is the significance of Breath 3?
A. This is an important breath as the abdomen holds stress. The psoas muscle[8] originates on the spine in the area of the abdomen. Air is also held in the gastrointestinal tract (the heaven element), as is food, the solid or earth element, and it contains fluids. The abdomen is really the meeting place of the physical components of body, soul and spirit. This is why it is called: *The Breath of Heaven and Earth.*

8 The psoas major muscle is an important muscle within the body and holds trauma. For more information on releasing trauma from this muscle see *Aranash Suba Yoga, The Yoga of Enlightenment.*

Q. The aphorism that accompanies Breath 3, Level I, states: *I embrace the changing expression of the fluid structure of my environment.* Can you expand on this?

A. We think we can find peace by holding onto static things. Peace is not found this way, but through the balance of movement and structure.

Q. The 4th breath is called *The Breath of the Little Horn.* To what does this refer?

A. A translation of the name is *Atma* (breath) *utu* (gate) *kranavesvi* (little horn) *uhut* (gate). The Little Horn refers to the coccyx bone – the tail bone. It is in the coccyx bone where most of the old garbage is kept – the old patterns that keep pulling us back into old behaviors even though we know we don't want to. It will also eliminate the programming of spirit, which dictates how we should live our lives and is a way to control physicality.[9] This is also held at the base of the spine.

Q. The aphorism to accompany Breath 4, Level 1 is: *I create my reality through the resonating emphases of my heart.*

A. In the film, *Don Juan de Marco,* the psychiatrist chose the fantasy reality as his own. In the movie *The Life of Pi,* the investigators and the authors choose the fantasy reality that the main character created. At the end, he asks them to choose which one is real. In actuality neither are real as there is no such thing as real. Reality is created. We create our reality by the song our heart wants to sing.

Q. You say that when the pranic tube is straightened, it will yield its full use as a grounding rod of man. What does this mean?

A. When the pranic tube is fully extended, it brings in the neutral energy of the Earth into the body. This is the very basis of health and peace. As a grounding rod, it also prevents cataclysmic change. This is why

9 See *Secrets of Dragon Magic, Sacred Fires of Hadji-ka.*

dragons and some ancient ones kept their tails. They wanted to keep it as a reminder of the importance of this part of the pranic tube.

Q. What is the intent of Breath 5 – *The Breath of the Fire Walk?*
A. There are chakras located in the arches of the feet. The purpose of walking on fire was to open these chakras. Although forgotten now, it was used in ancient times as a way of shocking these chakras into opening. The points below the feet, one hand length into the ground are also chakras. They are part of the body's 24 chakras (including the 12 chakras of the lower extremities that few know or teach about and have been unused).

Q. Why do we breathe in the left leg first?
A. The left leg is the feminine, receptive leg and receives from the Earth. The right leg is masculine and gives back to the Earth.

Q. Breath 6 is named *The Breath of the Divine Marriage*. Why is it so named?
A. A translation of the name – *Atma usu ama-uhet* – means the joining of masculine and feminine. This breath is the first time where you will find the complete, smooth interaction between the upper pranic tube and the lower pranic tube, between your life and death, between awake time and sleep time. As a result, the way you sleep will change. You will find wakefulness when you sleep and rest while you work.

Q. Can you elaborate on the aphorism for Breath 6 – *True peace is my constant companion through embracing unknowable change?*
A. Change is often only embraced if it is predictable. When we are comfortable with not knowing and allowing change to move, we will have achieved the deep peace of eternity.

Q. Can you tell us any more about Breath 6?

A. The breath follows the path of a figure 8 with the crossover point behind the navel. In physical life, the future lies in a loop in front of the navel and the past lies in a loop behind the navel (in a horizontal plane). The Mayans called this *'The Zuvuya'*. It is the loop or figure eight of time – time in physical life. In this way the future becomes the past and the past becomes the future as time moves through the point behind the belly button.

The upper part of the pranic tube, from the base of the spine to the crown, is used in life and it is from the crown that you exit at death. The lower part of the pranic tube, you live from when you are dead (the soul world) and you enter the body through the perineum while in utero. During these breaths, life and death are being combined.

The horizontal axis is physical life (body) and the vertical axis is soul and the breaths are also combining these 2 axes.

Q. When I was doing Breath 6, I also felt that as the crossover occurred behind the navel, it also happened in my nose. Can you explain this?

A. In the top of the nose, where the nose meets the forehead, is a point known as the gyroscope of the body. This breath works to combine space and spacelessness and it affects the gyroscope of the body in the nose, further evidence of the combining of the horizontal and vertical axes.

Q. Why is it important to eliminate the gaps between the in-breath and the out-breath in some of the breathing exercises?

A. Trauma is held in the gaps between the breaths and eliminating them aids in releasing the trauma.

In Breath 6, the cross over point for the change in the breaths occurs behind the belly button, the location of the life force center. Eliminating the gaps between the breaths at this point empowers the release of trauma. Initially it may be difficult to eliminate all the gaps between the breaths but with practice this should become easier. The more these gaps can be eliminated, the more trauma from life and death and from ascension and descension cycles can be released.

Q. What can you tell us about Breath 7?

A. This breath is amazing because for the first time there is actually cooperation between body, soul and spirit. The other breaths have created cooperation between body and soul. This means we are ending the war within and we cannot have peace until this is achieved.

When we speak of the triad of change, we talk about the body, soul and spirit. That is three points, but spirit actually has 2 points. Its other point is not on a flat plane. It is the point that creates a three-sided pyramid when the points are joined. This breath takes you off the flat disc of life into a three dimensional pyramid. What it does is create life not as a projection on a flat screen, but as a virtual reality.

It is the fountain of life because like the stem of a flower that is no longer cut, the pranic tube is no longer cut. The flow of energy no longer ends. It is a closed circuit, which means that your life becomes a self-sustaining energy device. This means that you no longer age, which is why it is called *'The Fountain of Life'*.

Q. The aphorism for Breath 7 is – *I love the totality of my experiences as the revelations of my greater self.* Can you elaborate on this?

A. We have spoken about how important self-love is for peace, but we also need self-acceptance. They can however, appear to be at war with and opposite to one another. The self is not the little self of the emotions, the thoughts and the body. The self is you throughout all your experiences – the greater self.

Yourself (the little self) is just the point in the center of the disc of life yet all you experience is you – it is your reality created by you. Self-acceptance also means accepting things in your environment. In the aphorism it states *'I love the totality of my experiences...'* not just some of my experiences because it is in the 'totality' that my greater self is revealed. It is only when we see things out of context that we view them as 'bad' or harmful or that we don't like them. Not liking them, we put a wall around them; separating them off as something we shouldn't be experiencing but only because we view them as separate from ourselves. We must become one with our environment.

Q. The out-breath of Breath 7 is the first time that the breath moves outside the body. Is there anything else we should know about this breath?

A. For the first time, there is no interruption of movement between the soul part of the pranic tube and the physical part of the pranic tube. These breaths cleanse the seven bodies of man and in Level I, Breath 7, we also work to cleanse the 4 directions.

In Level II, the breath moves out in a fountain in all directions as a full tube torus. It consists of trillions of yellow-gold light fibers. They are spirit's pranic tubes. Because man is the root race, the light fibers of the 7th body of man contain every other kingdom. Therefore every fiber in the tube torus represents life somewhere. As you do the 7th Breath, Level II, you are actually cleansing the kingdoms of existence.

This breath extends all the way up the entire pranic tube in a concentrated form and releases at the Lahun like a whale spout. This is significant as whales incorporate spirit and it is their song that puts the creational programs into things and this is also what spirit does for us in the original eight cells at the base of the spine.

Q. In Level II, Breath 1, the tip of the tongue presses against the roof of the mouth, why is this?

A. Pressing the tongue against the roof of the month releases more energy.

Q. The aphorism to accompany Breath 4, Level II states *"There is neither success nor failure upon the innocent journey of self-discovery.*

In the freedom of this knowledge, I explore life's revelations." Can you expand on this?

A. This is an important aphorism is relation to humility. Self-pity comes from people looking at their failures; self-importance comes from people looking at their successes. But there is neither success nor failure and this knowledge frees one up to just enjoy life and explore its revelations.

Q. Can you elaborate on the aphorism for Breath 6, Level II – *"Humility is not based on comparison, one thing being less than another, but by acknowledging the unknowableness of existence. True humility is the foundation of mastery."*

A. Life is unknowable. It is complete arrogance to think we know. *'I know nothing, I experience everything.'*

Q. In Level II when the breath travels through an area of the body, the color remains the same with the exception of when it travels down the right leg in Breath 6: instead of the color red, it is magenta. Why is this?

A. If the breath and energy were to remain red, it would overpower the orange on the left. Magenta balances the orange. Many people have had their courage to more forward in life broken by parents who said, *"don't do this, don't do that'*, by fearful circumstances *'no, it is not safe to do this or that'* or by having been ridiculed or feeling that they will be ridiculed.

Often people have broken meridians down the right leg. The red of Breath 5 re-establishes the function of the right leg as that which moves forward through life. Having established this, we now have magenta so that it balances with the orange of the left (receptive) leg.

The alchemical potency of red is to move forward or outward. Magenta contains some blue and blue contracts, giving a more measured movement through life. It provides a more contained, powerful movement, instead of a rushing-forward movement.

Q. In Breath 6, Level I, there is no gap between the out-breath and in-breath in the Lahun chakra, but a small gap as it transitions from the out-breath to the in-breath below the feet.

A. It is in the gaps that debris, old patterns and traumas are held and the breath can be powerfully purifying of the body. In Level I, because the gap in the Lahun chakra was closed, some detoxification and purification took place. To have closed both, the effect of the detoxification of the emotions and the body could have been overwhelming. Having practiced Level I for at least 5 days and released some debris, the gap at both the Lahun chakra and below the feet can be closed. Closing the gap at the Lahun chakra releases belief systems; closing the gap below the feet releases emotions.

Q. Having become the Fountain of Life (Breath 7), what does this really mean?

A. It means that you are actually going to be giving out an entirely new building block of life – one that is whole. Wherever you go, pollution can be cleared by your presence and effortless healing can come to those around you, even without intending it. It means that you have become life-giving because you are able to open the portal into infinite life which can only be opened within the still humility of your being. It requires body, soul and spirit and as you integrate this within yourself you are unlocking the key to eternal life. This is why it is called: The Seven Breaths of Eternal Life and The Breaths of the White Dove.[10]

---

10 It is also very powerful in enhancing the information contained in *Windows into Eternity.*

Appendix IV

Creating Sacred Space

Avoid interruptions of any sort as you create your sacred space and participate in your ceremony, whether it is a physical ceremony or one of intent. Once you start the ceremony it is best to complete it. Unplug the phone, go to the restroom, let others know that you wish to be undisturbed during this time.

Ceremonies build upon each other. It is recommended that they be completed in the order given. Ceremonies may be repeated as often as you feel is appropriate and right for you.

Note: Maintain the sacred space and circle. Keep animals and children out of the area by closing doors, etc. The frequency of the sacred circle is affected by their presence and they are affected by the ceremonial frequencies. These frequencies may be too high for them.

Recommendations during pregnancy: The frequencies of a ceremony may be too high for the baby and therefore, not comfortable. As a general rule, avoid doing ceremonies during pregnancy.

Working with Sacred Wheels

A wheel is a visual image that conveys non-cognitive, sacred and empowering information. They are similar to gateways through which specific healing frequencies are drawn and are power sources in the same way a holy object would be.

The wheels are alive and as we work with them they provide us with deep insights into the vastness and wealth of our own being, reminding us of all that we are.

Each wheel is a stand-alone wheel and can be used by itself. When wheels are used in a sequence, they tell a story and combine to make an equation.

Mystical practices have a beginning and a closure. If you are working with a sequence of wheels, do not stop in the middle as it leaks resources and energy. For this reason it is important that you always complete each sequence.

To access the information contained within the wheels at a deeper level you may place your hands on the wheels or run your hand across them – the left hand is receptive and the right hand promotes understanding. This technique may also be used for other sacred images, such as sigils and tablets, to access the deeper meaning contained within them.

Lying down, you may also place a wheel at your feet and upon contemplating its meaning, bring it up through your body from your feet to the Lahun Chakra, 10 inches above your head. If a wheel feels 'stuck' anywhere, continue to feel the quality of the wheel until it moves freely. If you are working with a sequence of wheels, ensure that the highest numbered wheel is at the bottom and the lowest numbered wheel is at the top. Work with one wheel at a time and fully integrate one before moving on to the next. As you do, also contemplate how the qualities of each wheel combine and complement the other wheels within the sequence.

Possible Uses for Wheels include:
- Meditate on a wheel.
- Place on the walls of a healing space, office or a room in which you spend a lot of time.
- With intention they can be placed into the body or placed directly on the body.

- Specific wheels can be placed under a healing table when working on someone or under a chair that you frequently sit on.
- Create your own personal mandala that you carry with you.

Other Books by Almine

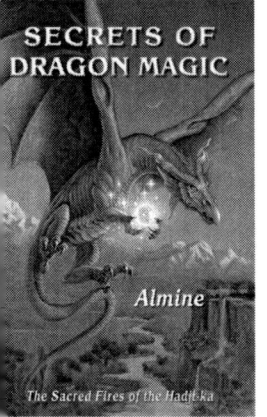

Secrets of Dragon Magic
The Sacred Fires of the Hadji-ka

This extraordinary record of the philosophy and practices of dragon magic is unmatched in its depth of knowledge and powerful delivery. From the *Sacred Records of the Hadji-ka*, kept by the dragons of Avondar, the secrets of Kundalini are revealed, designed to restore the innate, natural magical abilities of man lost by the separation of the spinal column and the pranic tube. The reader is swept along on a profound and mystical journey that pushes perception beyond mortal boundaries. Almine's infallible ability to empower her reading audience is clearly felt throughout the pages of this book.

Published: 2013, 418 pages, soft cover, 6 x 9, ISBN: 978-1-936926-56-5

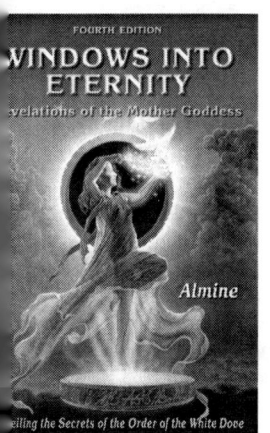

Windows into Eternity

Revelations of the Mother Goddess, 4th Edition

Through an unprecedented series of revelations, profound, upgraded material has been received by the Seer Almine to produce this powerful new edition.

This book provides unparalleled insight into ancient mysteries. The Seer Almine, an internationally recognized mystic and teacher, reveals the hidden laws of existence. Transcending reason and delivering visionary expansion, this metaphysical masterpiece explores the origins of life as recorded in the Holy Libraries. The release of information from these ancient libraries is a priceless gift to humankind.

Published 2013, 347 pages, soft cover, 6 x 9, ISBN: 978-1-936926-68-8

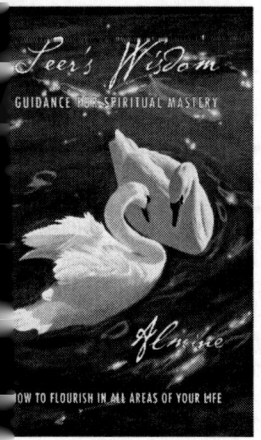

Seer's Wisdom
Guidance for Spiritual Mastery

Immerse yourself in the true nature of your being: Abundant living. This book shows you how to access your natural abundance and remove all blockages of flow. It is packed with over 400 pages of classic Almine aphorisms. Seer's Wisdom reminds you of the benign source of your own being and focuses your attention on attaining abundance: Abundance in yourself, abundance in your environment, abundance in your relationships and much more.

"To live within the Infinite's Being is to live in the fullness of an inexhaustible supply. Acknowledging the never-ending Source of abundance increases its accessibility."

Published: 2013, 430 pages, soft cover, 6 x 9, ISBN: 978-1-936926-52-7

Other Books by Almine

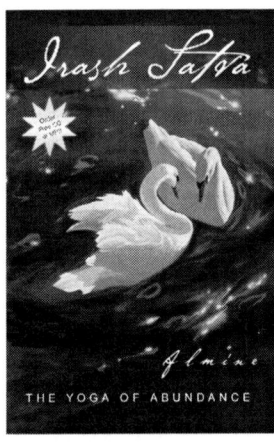

Irash Satva Yoga

Yoga, as a spiritual and physical discipline has been practiced in ma[n]
variations by masters and novices for countless years and is universal[ly]
accepted as one of the most effective development tools ever created.
Man's physical form in its original state was meant to be self-purifyin[g]
self-regenerating and self-transfiguring. Through pristine living a[nd]
total surrender, it was possible to open gates in the body that wou[ld]
allow life to permeate and flow through it; indefinitely sustaining it.
In Irash Satva Yoga, received by Almine from the Angelic Kingdo[m]
this ancient methodology is exponentially expanded and enhanced
incorporating the alchemies of sound and frequency.
Using easily mastered postures paired with music from Cosmic Sour[ce]
created specifically for each, the 144 cardinal gates in the mind a[nd]
body are opened and cleansed of their dross and debris, allowing [the]
practitioner to tap into the abundance of the One Life.

Published: 2010, 94 pages, soft cover, 6 x 9, ISBN: 978-1-934070-95[-]

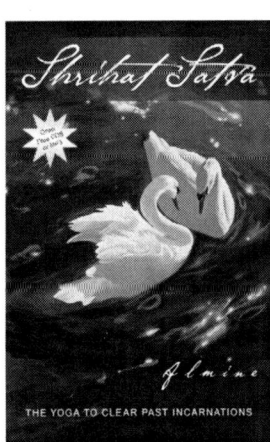

Shrihat Satva Yoga

The human body is unique in that it is an exact microcosm [of]
the macrocosm of created life. There are 12 points along [the]
right, masculine side of the body and the same number on t[he]
left side. These are microcosmic replicas of the macrocosm[ic]
cycles of life.
The yoga postures are designed to open and remove the deb[ris]
from these points – the gates of dreaming. This will occ[ur]
physically through the postures and the music. Dissolvi[ng]
debris also occurs by way of dreaming (triggered by [the]
breathing and eye movements), releasing past issues t[hat]
caused the blockages in the points

Published 2010, 108 pages, soft cover, 6 x 9, ISBN: 978-1-934070-1[5]

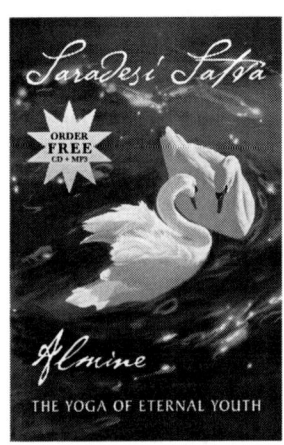

Saradesi Satva Yoga

The Yoga of Eternal Youth

As translated from the ancient texts of Saradesi – The Fount[ain]
of Youth. The ancient texts speak of time as moveme[nt]
They affirm that time and space, movement and stillne[ss]
are illusions. To sustain any illusion requires an enorm[ous]
amount of resources. This depletion of resources causes ag[ing]
and decay. The illusion of polarity, the impossibility that [the]
One Life can be divided and split is brought to resolut[ion]
by balancing the opposite poles exactly. Only then can t[hey]
cancel one another out, revealing an incorruptible reality t[hat]
lies beyond – the reality of Eternal Youth.

Published 2011, 115 pages, soft cover, 6 x 9, ISBN: 978-1-936926-0[2]

Other Books by Almine

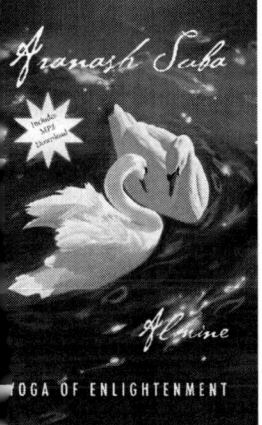

Aranash Suba Yoga - The Yoga of Enlightenment

Almine's yoga for releasing trauma and strengthening the Eternal Song of the Infinite within.

Aranash Suba Yoga works at a deep core level to assist with releasing trauma, specifically through the effects that the postures, meditations and stretches have on the psoas muscle. This yoga turns its back on the illusions of the matrices and embraces the contradiction of an existence of no opposites. The overall benefit of *Aranash Suba Yoga* is to release the hold of illusion and strengthen the Eternal Song of the Infinite within.

Published: 2012, 116 pages, soft cover, 6 x 9, ISBN: 978-1-936926-50-3

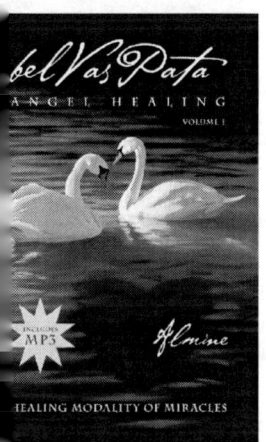

Belvaspata, Angel Healing, Volume I The Healing Modality of Miracles

Whether you are a beginner or an experienced master of the miraculous healing modality of Belvaspata, this comprehensive guide is an information rich handbook that will serve as your most valuable tool – a compendium of information for everything you need to know to establish yourself as a practitioner of this miraculous healing modality of the angels. Also included are Kaanish, Braamish Ananu and Song of the Self Belvaspata.

Published: 2011, 394 pages, soft cover, 6 x 9, ISBN: 978-1-936926-34-3

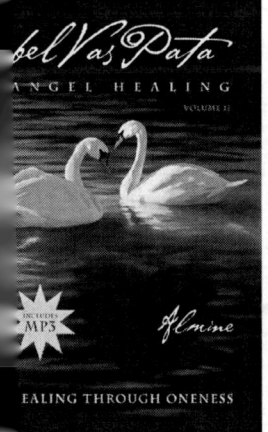

Belvaspata, Angel Healing, Volume 2 Healing through Oneness

Fairy Sound Elixir MP3 included

Whether you are a beginner or an experienced master of the miraculous healing modality of Belvaspata, this comprehensive guide is an information rich handbook that will serve as your most valuable tool – a compendium of information for everything you need to know to establish yourself as a practitioner of this miraculous healing modality of the angels. Belvaspata Volume II includes "The Integrated Use of Fragrance Alchemy," which delivers the method to obtain wellness of the emotional, mental and physical bodies through the combined use of Belvaspata, the alchemy of fragrance and the Atlantean Healing Sigils.

Published: 2012, 467 pages, soft cover, 6 x 9, ISBN: 978-1-936926-40-4

Other Books by Almine

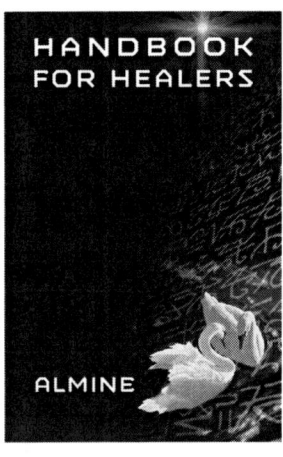

Handbook for Healers

The Healing Wisdom of the Seer Almine

Handbook for Healers is an invaluable tool for anyo
interested in self-healing or the healing of others. It offers bc
practical and spiritual guidance gleaned from the globa
acclaimed Seer Almine's advice to her students during the p:
decade. It reveals vital information on rejuvenating the bo
and understanding its communication through the language
pain, and many more empowering insights.

Published: 2013, 648 pages, soft cover, 6 x 9, ISBN: 978-1-936926-44-2

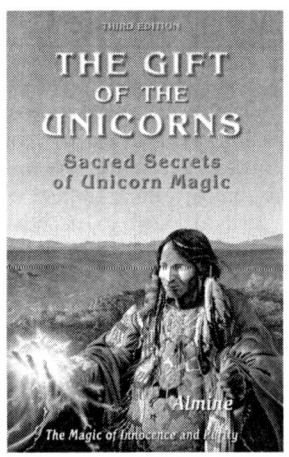

Gift of the Unicorns

Sacred Secrets of Unicorn Magic, 3rd Edition NEW

Where have the Unicorns gone? And, what about mysti
winged horses, mermaids, and giants – do they exist? 1
answers to all of our questions about these fabled creatu
can be found in The Gift of the Unicorns.
This magical book tells the story of the Unicorns and Pegas
and their heroism in preserving purity and innocence dur
the ages of darkness on Earth. In their own words, these bei
reveal where they went, the purpose of their golden sh
and the sacred mission they undertook for the Mother of
Creation. What's more, they share long-held secrets about
Earth.

Published: 2012, 188 pages, soft cover, 6 x 9, ISBN: 978-1-936926-48

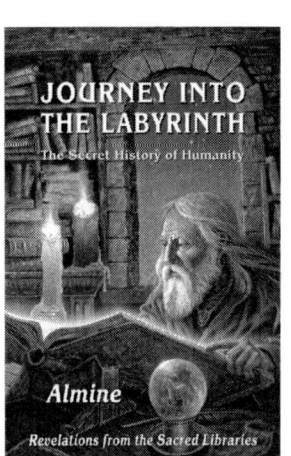

Journey Into the Labyrinth
Revelations from the Sacred Libraries

The online course *Revisiting the Labyrinth,* that has rive
truth-seekers from around the globe, is available now for
first time in book form. Disclosing the connection betw
the opening of hidden libraries and the awakening of the b
centers of man, this information packed book is bound to m
a life-changing impact.
Journey into the Labyrinth details the forgotten role of the E
and humanity, giving the reader new perspectives on the his
of our species. Drawing from records from the hidden sa
libraries of Earth, lost civilizations and the wisdoms preser
by the indigenous peoples of the Earth, this book revea
staggering older past then you may have ever imagined.

Published: 2012, 470 pages, soft cover, 6 x 9, ISBN: 978-1-936926-4

Other Books by Almine

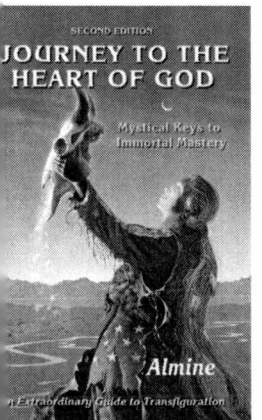

Journey to the Heart of God

Second Edition

Mystical Keys to Immortal Mastery

Ground-breaking cosmology revealed for the first time, sheds new light on previous bodies of information such as the Torah, the I Ching and the Mayan Zolkien. The explanation of man's relationship as the microcosm as set out in the previous book A Life of Miracles, is expanded in a way never before addressed by New Age authors, giving new meaning and purpose to human life. Endorsed by an Astro-physicist from Cambridge University and a former NASA scientist, this book is foundational for readers at all levels of spiritual growth.

Published: 2009, 276 pages, soft cover, 6 x 9, ISBN: 978-1-934070-26-0

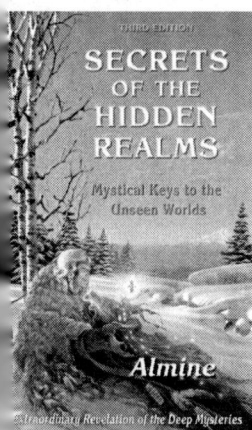

Secrets Of The Hidden Realms

Third Edition

Mystical Keys to the Unseen Worlds

This remarkable book delves into mysteries few mystics have ever revealed. It gives in detail:
- The practical application of the Goddess mysteries
- Secrets of the angelic realms
- The maps, alphabets, numerical systems of Lemuria, Atlantis, and the Inner Earth
- The Atlantean calender, accurate within 5 minutes
- The alphabet of the Akashic libraries.

Secrets of the Hidden Realms amazing bridge across the chasm that has separated humanity for eons from unseen realms.

Published: 2011, 412 pages, soft cover, 6 x 9, ISBN: 978-1-936926-38-1

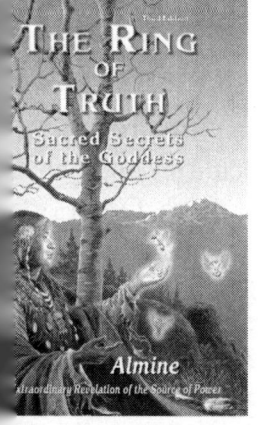

The Ring of Truth

Third Edition

Sacred Secrets of the Goddess

As man slumbers in awareness, the nature of his reality has altered forever. As one of the most profound mystics of all time, Almine explains this dramatic shift in cosmic laws that is changing life on earth irrevocably. A powerful healing modality is presented to compensate for the changes in the laws regarding energy that healers have traditionally relied upon. The new principles of beneficial white magic and the massive changes in spiritual warriorship are meticulously explained.

Published: 2009, 260 pages, soft cover, 6 x 9, ISBN: 978-1-934070-28-4

Music by Almine

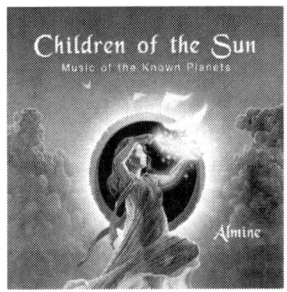

Children of the Sun

Music from the Known Planets (Re-mastered and re-titled version of the Interstellar Sound Elixirs) The beautiful interstellar sound elixirs received and sung by Almine.

Price $9.95 MP3 Download
$14.95 CD

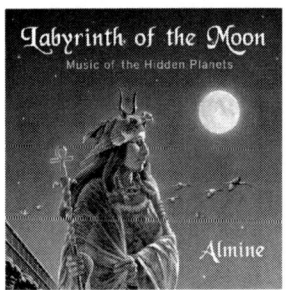

Labyrinth of the Moon

Music from the Hidden Planets (Re-titled version of the Sound Elixirs of the Hidden Planets) All the vocals in these elixirs are received and sung in the moment by Almine

Price $9.95 MP3 Download
$14.95 CD

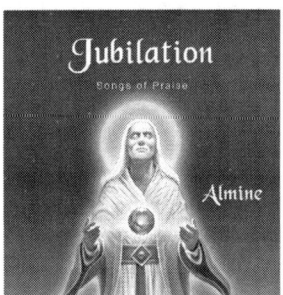

Jubilation – Songs of Praise

Music from around the world to lift the heart and inspire the listener. The extraordinary mystical quality of the music, and the exquisite clarity of Almine's voice, creates the ambient impression of being in the presence of angels.

Price $9.95 MP3 Download
$14.95 CD

Visit Almine's website www.spiritualjourneys com for worldwide retreat locations and dates online courses, radio shows and more. Order one Almine's many books, CDs or an instant downlo US toll-free phone: 1-877-552-5646